CRAM SESSION IN

Goniometry

A Handbook for Students & Clinicians

CRAM SESSION IN
Goniometry
A Handbook for Students & Clinicians

LYNN VAN OST, MEd, RN, PT, ATC
Hunterdon Medical Center
Flemington, NJ

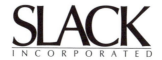

www.slackbooks.com

ISBN: 978-1-55642-898-2

The procedures and practices described in this book should be implemented in a manner consis-tent with the professional standards set for the circumstances that apply in each specific situation. Every effort has been made to confirm the accuracy of the information presented and to correctly relate generally accepted practices. The authors, editor, and publisher cannot accept responsibility for errors or exclusions or for the outcome of the material presented herein. There is no expressed or implied warranty of this book or information imparted by it. Care has been taken to ensure that drug selection and dosages are in accordance with currently accepted/recommended practice. Due to continuing research, changes in government policy and regulations, and various effects of drug reactions and interactions, it is recommended that the reader carefully review all materials and literature provided for each drug, especially those that are new or not frequently used. Any review or mention of specific companies or products is not intended as an endorsement by the author or publisher.

SLACK Incorporated uses a review process to evaluate submitted material. Prior to publication, educators or clinicians provide important feedback on the content that we publish. We welcome feedback on this work.

Published by: SLACK Incorporated
                6900 Grove Road
                Thorofare, NJ 08086 USA
                Telephone: 856-848-1000
                Fax: 856-848-6091
                www.slackbooks.com

Contact SLACK Incorporated for more information about other books in this field or about the availability of our books from distributors outside the United States.

Library of Congress Cataloging-in-Publication Data
Van Ost, Lynn.
Cram session in goniometry : a handbook for students & clinicians / Lynn Van Ost.
   p. ; cm.
Includes bibliographical references and index.
ISBN 978-1-55642-898-2 (alk. paper)
1. Joints--Range of motion--Measurement. 2. Angles (Geometry)--Measurement. I. Title.
[DNLM: 1. Arthrometry, Articular--methods--Handbooks. 2. Joints--physiology--Handbooks. 3. Patient Positioning--Handbooks. WE 39 V217c 2010]
RD734.V36 2010
617.4'72--dc22
                        2009051843

Printed in the United States of America.

Last digit is print number: 10   9   8   7   6   5   4   3   2   1

DEDICATION

To my parents, Marijane and Dr. William C. Van Ost, my stepmother, Elaine, and to my best friend, Karen Manfré, for their endless support and encouragement with all my endeavors.

CONTENTS

Dedication... v
Acknowledgments ix
About the Author.. xi
Preface...xiii

SECTION I: CERVICAL SPINE

The Cervical Spine 2

SECTION II: UPPER EXTREMITY

Scapulothoracic Joint 12
The Shoulder (Glenohumeral Joint) 20
The Elbow (Humeroulnar and Humeroradial Joints) 36
The Forearm (Radioulnar)... 40
The Wrist (Radiocarpal and Intercarpal Joints)............................. 44
The Fingers—Digits II to V (Metacarpophalangeal Joints)............ 52
The Fingers—Digits II to V (Proximal Interphalangeal Joints) 60
The Fingers—Digits II to V (Distal Interphalangeal Joints) 64
The Thumb (Carpometacarpal Joint) 68
The Thumb (Metacarpophalangeal Joint)....................................... 78
The Thumb (Interphalangeal Joint) 82

SECTION III: THORACIC AND LUMBAR SPINE

The Thoracolumbar Spine.. 88

SECTION IV: LOWER EXTREMITY

The Hip.. 98
The Knee (Tibiofemoral Joint) 110
Tibial Torsion 114
The Ankle 116
Subtalar Joint (Hindfoot)... 120
Transverse Tarsal (Midtarsal) Joint 124
The First Toe (Metatarsophalangeal Joints) 128
The First Toe (Interphalangeal Joint).. 134

The Four Lateral Toes (Metatarsophalangeal Joints)........................... 138

The Four Lateral Toes (Proximal Interphalangeal Joints)........................ 142

The Four Lateral Toes (Distal Interphalangeal Joints)............................ 146

SECTION V: TMJ JOINT

The Temporomandibular Joint.. 152

APPENDICES

Appendix A: General Procedure for Goniometric Measurement 160

Appendix B: Commonly Used Terms in Goniometry............................... 161

Appendix C: Normal Range of Motion Values in Adults 164

Appendix D: Anatomical Zero 168

Bibliography... 171

Index 173

ACKNOWLEDGMENTS

I would like to thank a number of individuals who have spent many hours assisting with the production of this book. To Michael Raymond, who served as the primary model for this book—this project could never have been completed without you. Thank you for your flexibility and professionalism during our photo sessions.

Thank you to Brian Lehrer, for once again modeling for my project—you always come through for me. My gratitude is also extended to Karen Manfré, Michelle Bartkowski, Jennifer Mintz, and Jenine LaFevere for many hours serving as the examiners in the photographs. Finally, another huge thank you goes out to Samantha M. Van Ost for spending numerous weekends and nights in front of the computer typing out the text for this manual and to Judd Strauss for being my "technical support." You guys are the best!

ABOUT THE AUTHOR

Lynn Van Ost, MEd, RN, PT, ATC, graduated in 1982 with a bachelor's degree in nursing from West Chester State College, West Chester, PA; NATABOC certified in athletic training in 1984; graduated in 1987 from Temple University, Philadelphia, PA, with a master's degree in sports medicine/athletic training; and received a second bachelor's degree in physical therapy in 1988 from Temple. In addition to treating the general orthopedic population as a physical therapist, she has worked with both amateur and professional athletes and has more than 11 years' experience as an athletic trainer working with Olympic-level elite athletes at numerous international events, including the 1992 and 1996 Summer Olympic games. She currently works as a clinical specialist in sports medicine at Hunterdon Medical Center in Flemington, NJ.

PREFACE

Although there are a number of published texts that include information regarding goniometric theory and application, there are few texts or manuals available that are solely dedicated to goniometric application and procedure. This manual was developed with the intent of addressing the "meat and potatoes" of goniometry. It does not address the theory of goniometry and does not support or refute its validity or reliability as a procedure for measuring the joints of the body. This manual is intended only as a user-friendly reference manual for the experienced clinician or student, not necessarily as a teaching tool or introductory text on the subject of goniometry. The target audience of this text is primarily physical therapists, occupational therapists, and athletic trainers, but its contents are valuable to all disciplines dealing with musculoskeletal disorders.

This text has been organized by body region in a "head to toe" fashion to make referencing easier and more efficient. Each region is broken down into a description of type of joint, capsular pattern, average range of motion for each movement, patient positioning, goniometric alignment, alternative methods of measurement, and patient substitutions. More than 190 photographs accompany the text, illustrating the initial and final position of the joint being measured, the goniometric alignment, alternative positioning, and patient substitutions. Although body part stabilization is described in the text, it is not always pictured to allow for better visualization of joint movement in the photographs. Also included in this book are four appendices describing procedure for measurement, goniometric terminology, average values of adult joint range of motion, and anatomical zero.

The author took care to present this manual in a clear, concise manner. If it makes the task of taking goniometric measurements during an examination easier and more accurate for the clinician, then the goal of this manual will have been achieved.

SECTION I

Cervical Spine

L. Van Ost
Cram Session in Goniometry:
A Handbook for Students & Clinicians (pp. 1-9)
© 2010 SLACK Incorporated

THE CERVICAL SPINE

Type of joint: The cervical spine is made up of a series of joints allowing for 3 degrees of freedom of the neck. The goniometer is only capable of measuring gross movements of the cervical spine; individual types of joints (eg, the atlantoccipital or atlantoaxial joints) will not be addressed in this section.

Capsular pattern: Lateral flexion = rotation/extension.

Cervical Flexion

Planes/axis of movement: Movement occurs in the sagittal plane around a coronal axis. It includes all segmental movements of the occiput, cervical, and thoracic vertebrae to approximately T7.

Range of motion:

- 0 degrees to 45 degrees with the goniometer

- 1.0 to 4.3 cm with tape measure

Preferred starting position: See Figure 1-1.

End position: See Figure 1-2.

Goniometric alignment:

- Axis: Center over the external auditory meatus

- Stationary arm: Align perpendicular to the floor

- Moving arm: Align parallel to the base of the nose

Stabilization: The trunk should be stabilized against the back of a chair.

Substitutions: The examiner must watch to make sure the subject does not flex the trunk or laterally bend/rotate the head during testing. These substitutions are commonly seen if the tested motion causes pain.

Alternate method/position for testing: See Figure 1-3.

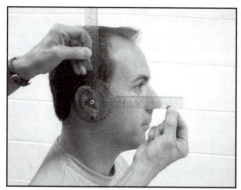

Figure 1-1. The subject should be sitting with the thoracic spine stabilized against a chair. The head is in neutral position. The hands should be in the subject's lap.

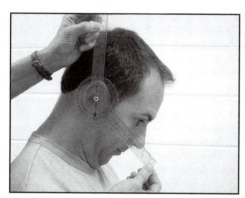

Figure 1-2. The cervical spine should be in a position of maximal flexion at the end of the movement.

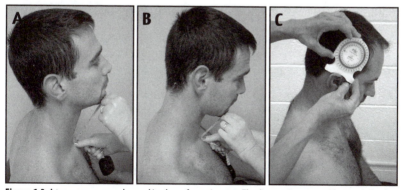

Figure 1-3. A tape measure may be used in place of a goniometer. The distance is measured between the chin and sternal notch. The subject's mouth should be closed during testing. (A) Alternate starting position. (B) End position. (C) A fluid goniometer may also be used with the base resting on top of the ear.

Cervical Extension/Hyperextension

Planes/axis of movement: Movement occurs in the sagittal plane around a coronal axis. It includes all segmental movements of the occiput, cervical, and thoracic vertebrae to approximately T7. Movement beyond neutral is considered hyperextension.

Range of motion:

- 45 degrees to 0 degrees of extension (from full flexion)
- 0 degrees to 45 degrees of hyperextension
- Approximately 7 inches of extension, using a tape measure
- Approximately 10 inches of hyperextension (from full flexion) using a tape measure

Preferred starting position: See Figure 1-4.

End position: See Figure 1-5.

Goniometric alignment:

- Axis: Center over the external auditory meatus
- Stationary arm: Align perpendicular to the floor
- Moving arm: Align parallel to the base of the nose

Stabilization: The trunk should be stabilized against the back of a chair.

Substitutions: The subject may try to extend the trunk or laterally bend/rotate the head during testing. These substitutions are commonly seen if the tested motion causes pain.

Alternate method/position for testing: See Figure 1-6.

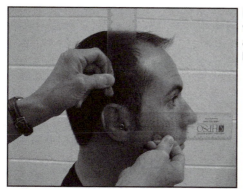

Figure 1-4. The subject should be sitting with the thoracic spine stabilized against a chair. The head is in neutral position. The hands should be in the subject's lap.

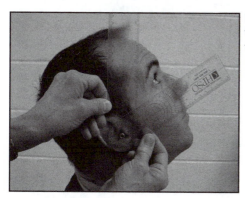

Figure 1-5. The cervical spine should be in full cervical extension/hyperextension at the end of the movement.

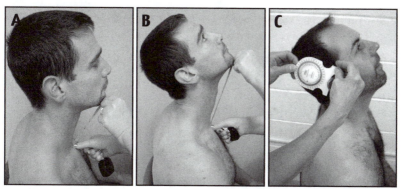

Figure 1-6. A tape measure may be used in place of a goniometer. The distance is measured between the chin and the sternal notch. (A) Alternate starting position. (B) End position. (C) A fluid goniometer may also be used with the base resting on top of the ear.

Cervical Lateral Flexion

Planes/axis of movement: Movement occurs in the frontal plane around an anterior/posterior axis and occurs segmentally along the cervical vertebrae. There is a component of rotation that occurs to allow for full movement of the head.

Range of motion:

- 0 degrees to 45 degrees
- Approximately 5 inches if using a tape measure

Preferred starting position: See Figure 1-7.

End position: See Figure 1-8.

Goniometric alignment:

- Axis: Center over the spinous process of C7
- Stationary arm: Align perpendicular to the floor
- Moving arm: Align over the external occipital protuberance of the occiput

Stabilization: The trunk should be stabilized against the back of a chair. Additional stabilization is achieved by holding the subject's shoulder down with the clinician's hand.

Substitutions: The subject may try to laterally flex the trunk or rotate the head to increase the range of motion or avoid pain with movement.

Alternate method/position for testing: See Figure 1-9.

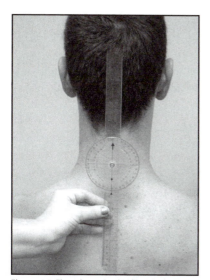

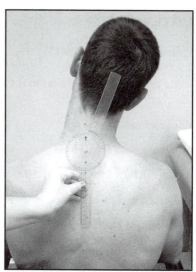

Figure 1-7. The subject should be sitting with the thoracic spine stabilized against a chair. The head is in a neutral position. The hands should be in the subject's lap.

Figure 1-8. The cervical spine should be in full lateral cervical flexion at the end of the movement.

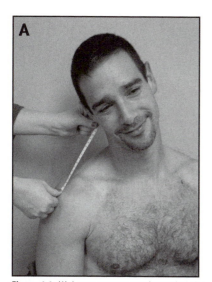

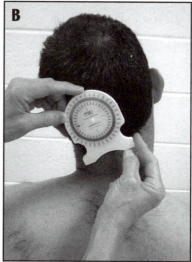

Figure 1-9. (A) A tape measure may be used in place of a goniometer. The distance between the mastoid process and acromion process is measured. It is important to measure and record the differences in length between the starting position and end position in determining the range of motion. (B) A fluid goniometer may also be used with the base aligned with the external occipital protuberance.

Cervical Rotation

Planes/axis of movement: Movement occurs in the transverse plane around a vertical axis. Most of this motion occurs at the atlantoaxial joint (C1-C2). Some cervical lateral flexion to the same side of the rotation should occur during movement.

Range of motion:

- 0 degrees to 60 degrees

- Approximately 5 inches if using a tape measure

Preferred starting position: See Figure 1-10.

End position: See Figure 1-11.

Goniometric alignment:

- Axis: Align over the center of the top of the head

- Stationary arm: Align with the acromion process of the tested side

- Moving arm: Align with the tip of the nose

Stabilization: The trunk should be stabilized against the back of a chair.

Substitutions: The subject may try to rotate the trunk, laterally flex the neck, or elevate the scapula to the tested side to avoid pain during the movement.

Alternate method/position for testing: See Figure 1-12.

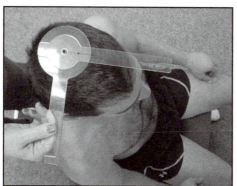

Figure 1-10. The subject should be in sitting with the head in neutral position and the hands in the subject's lap.

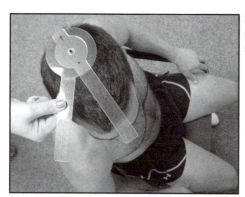

Figure 1-11. The cervical spine should be in full cervical rotation at the end of the movement.

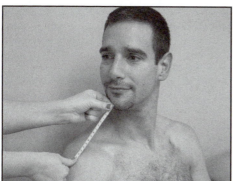

Figure 1-12. A tape measure may be used in place of a goniometer. The distance between the top of the chin and the same side acromion process is measured. It is important to measure and record the differences in length between the starting position and end position in determining the range of motion.

SECTION II

Upper Extremity

L. Van Ost
Cram Session in Goniometry:
A Handbook for Students & Clinicians (pp. 11-85)
© 2010 SLACK Incorporated

SCAPULOTHORACIC JOINT

Type of joint: Movements relating to the scapula sliding over the thorax are described as movements of the scapulothoracic joint. This is a "functional" joint in which there are no typical joint characteristics. All movements of the scapula and scapulothoracic joint are intimately related to the sternoclavicular and acromioclavicular joints, but these joint articulations will not be discussed as they cannot be measured with a goniometer. The best method for determining scapulothoracic joint movement is by the use of a tape measure.

Capsular pattern: None.

Scapular Upward Rotation

Planes/axis of movement: Motion occurs in the frontal plane around an anterior/posterior axis during glenohumeral abduction and flexion. The inferior angle of the scapula moves away from the vertebral column.

Range of motion:

- Normal range of motion is determined by comparing the motion of one scapula to the other. The measurement is recorded in inches or centimeters between the anatomical starting and ending positions.

Preferred starting position: See Figure 2-1.

End position: See Figure 2-2.

Goniometric alignment points: The inferior angle of the scapula and the spinous process of the seventh thoracic vertebra T7 are palpated and identified.

Measurement of motion: The distance between the inferior angle of the scapula and the spinous process of the seventh thoracic vertebra T7 is measured. The subject fully abducts the shoulder and a second measurement is taken. The difference between the two measurements is the amount of scapular upward rotation present.

Stabilization: Thoracic stabilization is achieved through subject compliance.

Substitutions: The subject may attempt to laterally flex or extend the trunk to gain more shoulder motion. This may be more commonly seen in individuals with upper extremity weakness or those with glenohumeral limitations.

Alternate method/position for testing: See Figure 2-3.

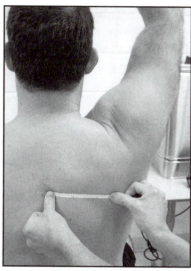

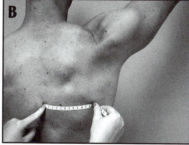

Figure 2-1. The subject should sit with the shoulder in anatomical position. The upper extremity should be in a neutral position.

Figure 2-2. The shoulder is maximally abducted or flexed to allow for full scapular upward rotation.

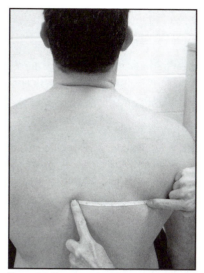

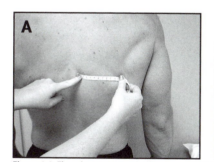

Figure 2-3. The subject may stand or lie prone. (A) Alternate starting position. (B) End position.

Scapular Downward Rotation

Planes/axis of movement: Motion occurs in the frontal plane around an anterior/posterior axis. Downward rotation of the scapula is a rotary movement of the inferior angle toward the vertebral column. It occurs during shoulder adduction and extension across the posterior trunk.

Range of motion:

- Normal range of motion is determined by comparing the motion of one scapula to the other. The measurement is recorded in inches or centimeters between the anatomical starting position and ending position.

Preferred starting position: See Figure 2-4.

End position: See Figure 2-5.

Goniometric alignment points: The inferior angle of the scapula and the spinous process of the T7 vertebra are palpated and identified.

Measurement of motion: The distance between the inferior angle of the scapula and the spinous process of T7 is measured. The subject fully adducts the upper limb across the posterior trunk and a second measurement is taken. The difference between the two measurements is the amount of scapular downward rotation present.

Stabilization: Thoracic stabilization is achieved through subject compliance.

Substitutions: The subject may try to retract the scapula to gain more motion. This may be seen in individuals with range of motion limitations at the glenohumeral joint.

Alternate method/position for testing: See Figure 2-6.

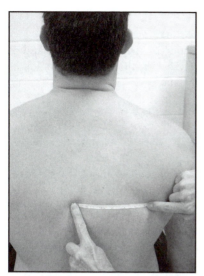 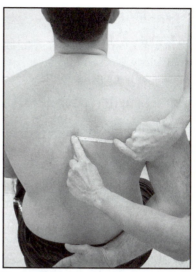

Figure 2-4. The subject should sit with the shoulder in anatomical position. The upper extremity should be in a neutral position.

Figure 2-5. The subject is asked to maximally extend and adduct his/her arm across his/her back.

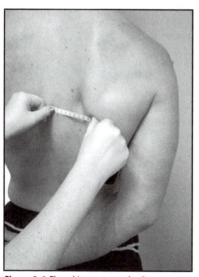

Figure 2-6. The subject may stand or lie prone.

Scapular Abduction

Planes/axis of movement: Motion occurs in the frontal plane and is translatory. The scapula moves laterally across the thorax as the shoulder is horizontally adducted in the transverse plane.

Preferred starting position: See Figure 2-7.

End position: See Figure 2-8.

Goniometric alignment points: The origin or "root" of the spine of the scapula is palpated and identified. The corresponding thoracic vertebra at that level is also palpated and identified.

Measurement of motion: The distance between the origin of the spine of the scapula and the thoracic vertebrae is measured. The subject fully horizontally adducts the shoulder across the anterior trunk and a second measurement is taken. The difference between the two measurements is the amount of scapular abduction present.

Stabilization: Thoracic stabilization is achieved through subject compliance.

Substitutions: The examiner must be aware of the individual trying to rotate the glenohumeral joint or laterally flex the trunk to gain more motion or avoid pain during the motion.

Alternate method/position for testing: None.

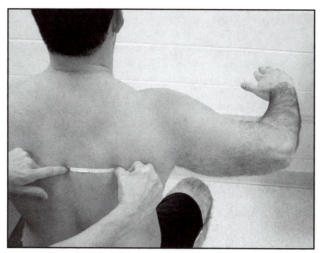

Figure 2-7. The subject should be sitting with the shoulder in 90 degrees of abduction. The elbow should be flexed to 90 degrees; the forearm and wrist should be in neutral positions.

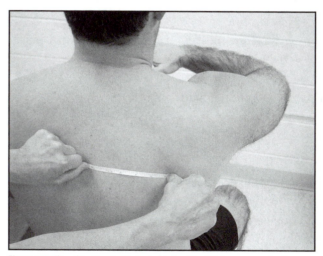

Figure 2-8. The subject is asked to horizontally adduct his/her arm maximally across his/her chest.

Scapular Adduction

Planes/axis of movement: Motion occurs in the frontal plane and is translatory. The scapula moves medially across the thorax as the shoulder is horizontally abducted in the transverse plane.

Preferred starting position: See Figure 2-9.

End position: See Figure 2-10.

Goniometric alignment points: The origin or "root" of the spine of the scapula is palpated and identified. The corresponding thoracic vertebra at that level is also palpated and marked.

Measurement of motion: The distance between the origin of the spine of the scapula and the thoracic vertebrae is measured. The subject fully horizontally abducts the shoulder across the posterior trunk and a second measurement is taken. The difference between the two measurements is the amount of scapular adduction present.

Stabilization: Thoracic stabilization is achieved through subject compliance.

Substitutions: The examiner must be aware of the individual trying to rotate the shoulder joint or rotate the trunk to gain more motion or avoid pain during the movement.

Alternate method/position for testing: None.

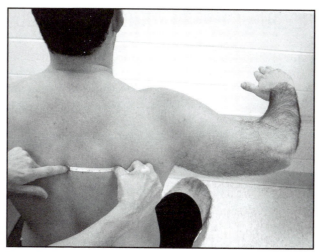

Figure 2-9. The subject should be sitting with the shoulder in 90 degrees of abduction. The elbow should be flexed to 90 degrees; the forearm and wrist should be in neutral positions.

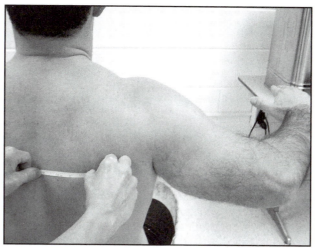

Figure 2-10. The subject is asked to maximally horizontally abduct his/her shoulder across the posterior thorax.

THE SHOULDER (GLENOHUMERAL JOINT)

Type of joint: Ball and socket joint with three degrees of freedom allowing for flexion/extension, abduction/adduction, and internal/external rotation. The anatomic axis is through the center of the head of the humerus.

Capsular pattern: Internal rotation > abduction > external rotation.

Shoulder Flexion

Planes/axis of movement: Motion occurs in the sagittal plane around a transverse axis through the head of the humerus.

Range of motion:

■ 0 degrees to 180 degrees

Preferred starting position: See Figure 2-11.

End position: See Figure 2-12.

Goniometric alignment:

■ Axis: Near the acromion process, through the humeral head

■ Stationary arm: Align with the midaxillary line of the trunk

■ Moving arm: Align with the lateral midline of the humerus siting the lateral epicondyle of the humerus

Stabilization: The scapula must be stabilized against a supporting surface by the weight of the trunk to prevent elevation, upward rotation, and posterior tilting. The clinician may use his/her hand to stabilize the scapula if the subject is in sitting.

Substitutions: Common substitutions in an attempt to gain more shoulder flexion may include lumbar hyperextension, shoulder abduction, or scapular elevation. These substitutions may occur because of limitations at the glenohumeral joint or as a result of pain during testing.

Alternate method/position for testing: See Figure 2-13.

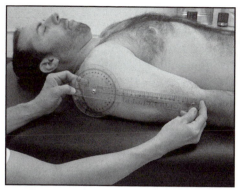

Figure 2-11. The subject is positioned in supine with the knees flexed to stabilize the lumbar spine. The elbow is extended and the forearm is in midposition between supination and pronation.

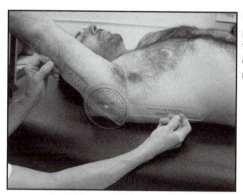

Figure 2-12. The shoulder should be in a position of maximal flexion at the end of the movement. The elbow should be in extension and the forearm should be in a neutral position.

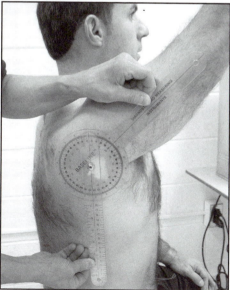

Figure 2-13. The subject may be placed in sitting.

Shoulder Extension/Hyperextension

Planes/axis of movement: Motion occurs in the sagittal plane around a transverse axis through the head of the humerus. Extension is the reverse action of flexion. As the arm passes the trunk in the anatomic position, hyperextension occurs.

Range of motion:

- 180 degrees to 0 degrees of extension (from full flexion)
- 0 degrees to 40 to 60 degrees of hyperextension

Preferred starting position: See Figure 2-14.

End position: See Figure 2-15.

Goniometric alignment:

- Axis: Near the acromion process, through the humeral head
- Stationary arm: Align with the midaxillary line of the trunk
- Moving arm: Align with the lateral midline of the humerus siting the lateral epicondyle of the humerus

Stabilization: The scapula should be stabilized against a supporting surface by the weight of the trunk to prevent anterior tilting and elevation. The clinician may use his/her hand to stabilize the scapula if the subject is in sitting.

Substitutions: The subject may try to extend the trunk or abduct the shoulder to complete the motion or avoid pain during testing.

Alternate method/position for testing: See Figure 2-16.

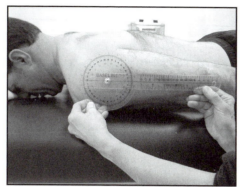

Figure 2-14. The subject is placed in the prone position with the forearm in midposition between supination and pronation. The head should not be supported by a pillow and the elbow should be slightly flexed.

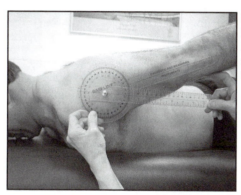

Figure 2-15. The shoulder should be in a position of maximal extension/hyperextension at the end of the movement. The elbow should be in extension with the forearm in a pronated position.

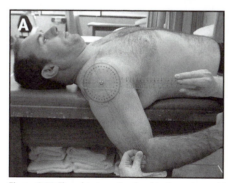

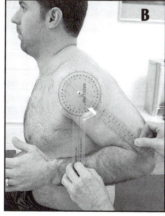

Figure 2-16. The subject may be placed in the supine position (A) with the arm resting over the side of the table, in sidelying or in sitting (B).

Shoulder Abduction

Planes/axis of movement: Motion occurs in the frontal plane around an anterior/posterior axis.

Range of motion:

- 0 degrees to 180 degrees

Preferred starting position: See Figure 2-17.

End position: See Figure 2-18.

Goniometric alignment:

- Axis: Close to the anterior aspect of the acromion process through the center of the humeral head
- Stationary arm: Align parallel to the midline of the sternum along the lateral aspect of the trunk
- Moving arm: Align along the medial midline of the humerus siting the medial epicondyle of the humerus

Stabilization: The scapula must be stabilized against a supporting surface by the weight of the trunk. The clinician may also use his/her hand to stabilize the clavicle and scapula if necessary to prevent elevation and upward rotation.

Substitutions: The examiner should not allow the subject to elevate the scapula or laterally flex the trunk to the contralateral side during testing in an attempt to gain more range of motion. Allow the shoulder to externally rotate during testing.

Alternate method/position for testing: See Figure 2-19.

Goniometric alignment if testing in sitting:

- Axis: Posterior aspect of the acromion process, through the center of the humeral head
- Stationary arm: Align parallel to the spinous process of the vertebral column
- Moving arm: Align on the posterior aspect of the humeral shaft, siting the olecranon process of the ulna

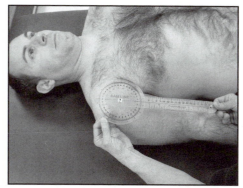

Figure 2-17. The subject should be placed in the supine position. The shoulder should be in midposition between flexion and extension with the shoulder in full external rotation. The forearm should be in midposition between supination and pronation with the elbow in full extension.

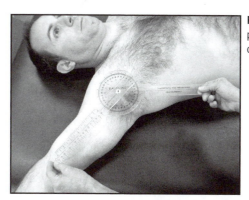

Figure 2-18. The shoulder should be in a position of maximal abduction at the end of the movement.

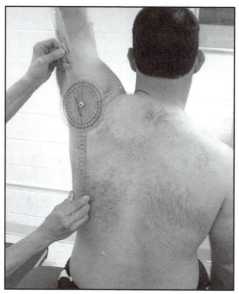

Figure 2-19. The subject may be placed in a prone or sitting position.

Shoulder Adduction

Planes/axis of movement: Movement occurs in the frontal plane around an anterior/posterior axis. It is discontinued by contact of the upper arm with the body.

Range of motion:

- 180 degrees to 0 degrees (from full abduction)

Preferred starting position: See Figure 2-20.

End position: See Figure 2-21.

Goniometric alignment:

- Axis: Anterior aspect of the acromion process, through the center of the humeral head

- Stationary arm: Align along the lateral aspect of the anterior surface of the trunk in parallel with the midline of the sternum

- Moving arm: Align with the midline of the humerus siting the medial epicondyle of the humerus

Stabilization: Stabilize the thorax against a supporting surface and encourage subject compliance to prevent ipsilateral flexion. Allow the shoulder to internally rotate.

Substitutions: The subject may try to laterally flex the trunk toward the tested side to gain more motion or avoid pain during testing.

Alternate method/position for testing: The subject may be placed in a sitting position.

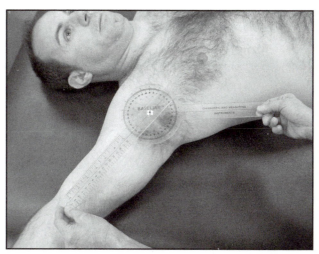

Figure 2-20. Subject lies supine with the shoulder in a maximally abducted and externally rotated position.

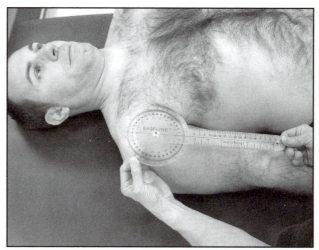

Figure 2-21. The upper extremity should come to rest at the maximum range of shoulder adduction.

Shoulder Horizontal Abduction

Planes/axis of movement: Movement occurs in the transverse plane around a vertical axis. The scapula adducts on the thorax during movement.

Range of motion:

- 0 degrees to 45 degrees from neutral
- 0 degrees to 135 degrees from a fully horizontally adducted position

Preferred starting position: See Figure 2-22.

End position: See Figure 2-23.

Goniometric alignment:

- Axis: The superior aspect of the acromion process through the head of the humerus
- Stationary arm: Align along the midline of the shoulder siting the base of the neck
- Moving arm: Align along the midline of the humeral shaft, siting the lateral epicondyle of the humerus

Stabilization: The thorax must be stabilized against the back of a chair to prevent trunk rotation.

Substitutions: The subject may attempt to rotate the trunk or laterally flex to the opposite side to gain more movement. Scapular elevation is also another substitution seen during testing.

Alternate method/position for testing: None.

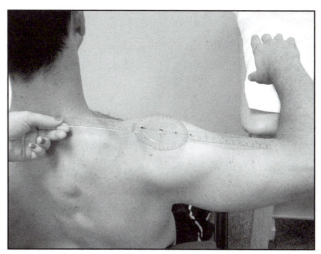

Figure 2-22. The subject should be sitting with the shoulder in neutral rotation. The shoulder should be abducted to 90 degrees with the elbow in 90 degrees of flexion.

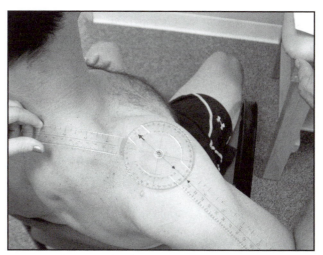

Figure 2-23. The shoulder should be in a position of maximal horizontal abduction with the scapula fully adducted.

Shoulder Horizontal Adduction

Planes/axis of movement: Movement occurs in the transverse plane around a vertical axis. The scapula abducts on the thorax during the movement.

Range of motion:

- 0 degrees to 90 degrees from neutral

- 0 degrees to 135 degrees from a fully horizontally abducted position

Preferred starting position: See Figure 2-24.

End position: See Figure 2-25.

Goniometric alignment:

- Axis: The superior aspect of the acromion process of the scapula, through the head of the humerus

- Stationary arm: Align along the midline of the shoulder siting the base of the neck

- Moving arm: Align along the midline of the humeral shaft, siting the lateral epicondyle of the humerus

Stabilization: The thorax must be stabilized against the back of a chair or supporting surface to prevent rotation.

Substitutions: The subject may try to rotate the trunk to obtain more motion during testing.

Alternate method/position for testing: See Figure 2-26.

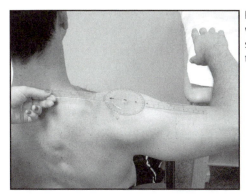

Figure 2-24. The subject should be sitting with the shoulder in neutral rotation. The shoulder joint is flexed to 90 degrees and the elbow is flexed to 90 degrees.

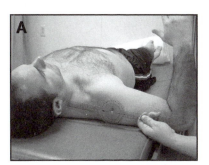

Figure 2-25. The shoulder should be in a position of maximal horizontal adduction at the end of the movement.

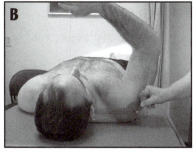

Figure 2-26. The subject lies in supine with the shoulder joint in 90 degrees abduction and neutral rotation and with the elbow in 90 degrees of flexion. (A) Alternate starting position. (B) End position.

Shoulder Internal (Medial) Rotation

Planes/axis of movement: Movement occurs in the transverse plane around a longitudinal axis through the head and shaft of the humerus.

Range of motion:

- With the shoulder stabilized: 0 degrees to 75 degrees
- Universally accepted range of motion: 0 degrees to 90 degrees

Preferred starting position: See Figure 2-27.

End position: See Figure 2-28.

Goniometric alignment:

- Axis: Over the olecranon process of the ulna
- Stationary arm: Align perpendicular to the floor
- Moving arm: Align with the shaft of the ulna, siting the styloid process of the ulna

Stabilization: Make sure the distal end of the humeral shaft is stabilized against a supporting surface and the trunk does not rise during the movement.

Substitutions: The trunk or anterior shoulder may elevate to accommodate a restricted joint capsule. The subject may also adduct or extend either the shoulder or elbow to avoid internally rotating the shoulder.

Alternate method/position for testing: See Figure 2-29.

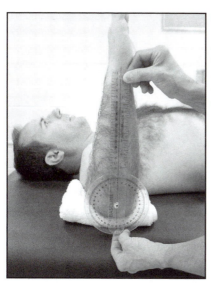

Figure 2-27. The subject should be in supine, with the shoulder joint positioned in 90 degrees of abduction. The forearm is placed in midposition between supination and pronation. The palm faces down toward the floor. The humerus is placed level with the acromion process by placing a pad under the upper arm. The elbow rests off the table.

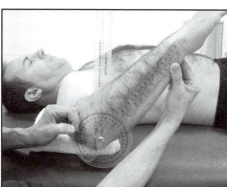

Figure 2-28. The shoulder should be in maximal internal rotation at the end of the movement with the palm facing the floor.

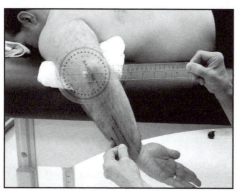

Figure 2-29. The subject may be placed in the prone position with the shoulder in 90 degrees abduction and with the elbow flexed to 90 degrees over the edge of the table.

Shoulder External (Lateral) Rotation

Planes/axis of movement: Motion occurs in the transverse plane around a longitudinal axis through the head and shaft of the humerus.

Range of motion:

- 0 degrees to 90 degrees

Preferred starting position: See Figure 2-30.

End position: See Figure 2-31.

Goniometric alignment:

- Axis: Over the olecranon process of the ulna
- Stationary arm: Align perpendicular to the floor
- Moving arm: Align with the shaft of the ulna, siting the styloid process of the ulna

Stabilization: Make sure the distal end of the humerus is stabilized against a supporting surface and the trunk does not rise during movement.

Substitutions: The examiner should watch carefully to make sure the subject does not extend the trunk or move the shoulder out of 90 degrees of abduction to avoid the movement. Elbow flexion or extension is another commonly seen substitution to avoid shoulder external rotation.

Alternate method/position for testing: The subject is in the prone position with the shoulder abducted to 90 degrees and the elbow flexed to 90 degrees over the edge of the table.

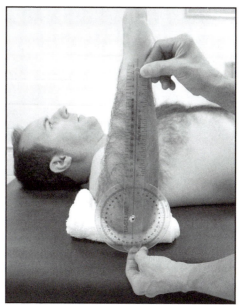

Figure 2-30. The subject should be lying in supine with the shoulder positioned in 90 degrees of abduction. The forearm is placed in midposition between supination and pronation. The palm faces down toward the floor. The humerus is placed level with the acromion process by placing a pad under the upper arm. The elbow rests off the table.

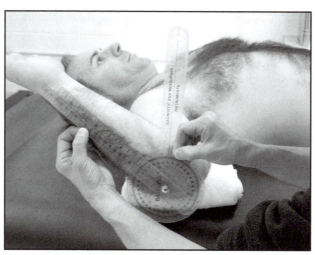

Figure 2-31. The shoulder should be in a position of maximal external rotation at the end of the movement.

THE ELBOW (HUMEROULNAR AND HUMERORADIAL JOINTS)

Type of joint: Hinge joint (ginglymus) with one degree of freedom allowing for flexion and extension.

Capsular pattern: Flexion > extension.

Elbow Flexion

Planes/axis of movement: Motion occurs in the sagittal plane around a coronal axis.

Range of motion:

- 0 degrees to 145 degrees

Preferred starting position: See Figure 2-32.

End position: See Figure 2-33.

Goniometric alignment:

- Axis: Over the lateral epicondyle of the humerus
- Stationary arm: Align along the lateral midline of the humerus, siting the acromion process
- Moving arm: Align along the lateral midline of the radius, siting the radial styloid

Stabilization: The distal end of the humerus should be stabilized against a supporting surface to prevent shoulder flexion.

Substitutions: See Figure 2-34.

Alternate method/position for testing: None.

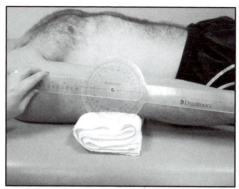

Figure 2-32. The subject lies supine with the upper arm close to the body. The shoulder should be in neutral position between flexion and extension. The forearm should be in supination. A pad should be placed at the distal end of the humerus to allow for full motion.

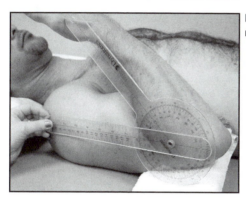

Figure 2-33. The elbow should be in maximal flexion at the end of the movement.

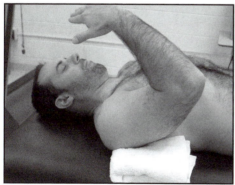

Figure 2-34. The subject may attempt to flex the shoulder to avoid pain or pronate the forearm to gain more motion during testing.

Elbow Extension

Planes/axis of movement: Movement occurs in the sagittal plane around a coronal axis.

Range of motion:

- 145 degrees to 0 degrees

Preferred starting position: See Figure 2-35.

End position: See Figure 2-36.

Goniometric alignment:

- Axis: On the lateral epicondyle of the humerus
- Stationary arm: Align along the lateral midline of the humerus, siting the acromion process
- Moving arm: Align along the lateral midline of the radius, siting the radial styloid

Stabilization: The proximal humerus should be stabilized anteriorly by the clinician's hand to prevent scapular protraction and trunk extension.

Substitutions: The subject may try to extend the trunk to enhance the motion or move the shoulder into flexion or extension to avoid pain with testing.

Alternate method/position for testing: None.

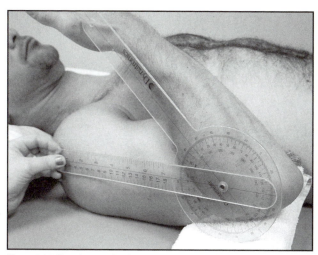

Figure 2-35. The subject is placed in a supine position with the upper arm alongside the trunk with the forearm in full supination and with the elbow maximally flexed.

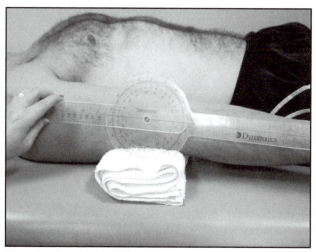

Figure 2-36. The elbow should be in maximal extension at the end of the move-ment.

THE FOREARM (RADIOULNAR)

Type of joint: The proximal radioulnar joint may be considered alone as a uniaxial pivot joint with one degree of freedom.

Capsular pattern: Pronation = supination.

Forearm Pronation

Planes/axis of movement: Motion occurs in the transverse plane around a longitudinal axis in the anatomical position. Motion occurs in the frontal plane while in the preferred testing position.

Range of motion:

- 0 degrees to 90 degrees

Preferred starting position: See Figure 2-37.

End position: See Figure 2-38.

Goniometric alignment:

- Axis: Lateral to the ulnar styloid
- Stationary arm: Align parallel to the anterior midline of the humerus
- Moving arm: Align across the dorsal aspect of the wrist, proximal to the styloid process of the ulna and radius

Stabilization: The distal end of the humerus must be stabilized on a supporting surface to prevent internal rotation and abduction at the shoulder joint. The subject may use the nontested hand to keep the humeral shaft against the thorax.

Substitutions: The subject may try to laterally flex the trunk away from the tested side or abduct/internally rotate the shoulder to increase the amount of range of motion.

Alternate method/position for testing: See Figure 2-39.

Goniometric alignment for alternate method:

- Axis: The third metacarpal head, siting through the third metacarpal shaft
- Stationary arm: Align perpendicular to the table surface
- Moving arm: Align parallel to the midline of the pencil

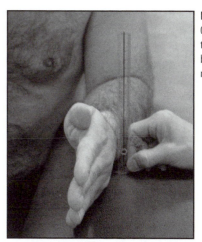

Figure 2-37. The subject is sitting with the shoulder in 0 degrees of abduction, flexion, and extension and with the elbow flexed to 90 degrees. The forearm should be in midposition between pronation and supination resting on a tabletop.

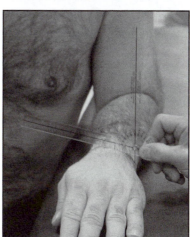

Figure 2-38. The forearm should be in a position of maximal pronation at the end of the movement.

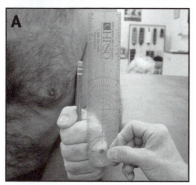
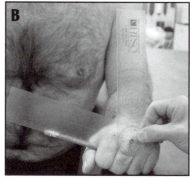

Figure 2-39. The subject may be in sitting gripping a pencil or pen vertically in his/her hand. (A) Alternate starting position. (B) End position.

Forearm Supination

Planes/axis of movement: Movement occurs in the transverse plane around a longitudinal axis in the anatomical position. Motion occurs in the frontal plane while in the preferred testing position.

Range of motion:

- 0 degrees to 90 degrees

Preferred starting position: See Figure 2-40.

End position: See Figure 2-41.

Goniometric alignment:

- Axis: Center medial to the ulnar styloid process

- Stationary arm: Align on the anterior surface of the wrist parallel to the anterior midline of the humerus

- Moving arm: Place on the ventral surface of the wrist, just proximal to the styloid process of the ulna and radius

Stabilization: The humerus must be stabilized on a supporting surface to prevent external rotation of the shoulder. The subject may use the nontested hand to keep the humeral shaft against the thorax.

Substitutions: The subject may try to use shoulder external rotation to avoid a painful motion. The examiner may also observe the subject laterally flexing to the tested side or extending the elbow to obtain more movement.

Alternate method/position for testing: See Figure 2-42.

Goniometric alignment for alternate method:

- Axis: The third metacarpal head, siting through the third metacarpal shaft

- Stationary arm: Align perpendicular to the table surface

- Moving arm: Align parallel to the midline of the pencil

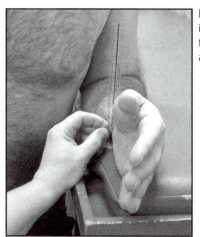

Figure 2-40. The subject is sitting with the shoulder in 0 degrees abduction, flexion, and extension. The forearm is placed in midposition between supination and pronation, resting on a tabletop.

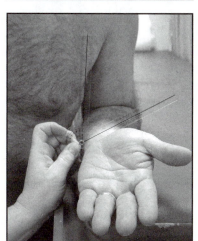

Figure 2-41. The forearm should be in a position of maximal supination at the end of the motion.

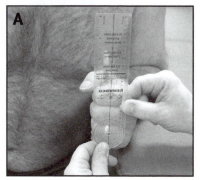
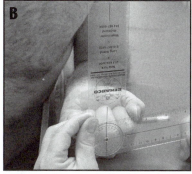

Figure 2-42. The subject may be in a sitting position gripping a pencil or pen vertically in his/her hand. (A) Alternate starting position. (B) End position.

THE WRIST
(RADIOCARPAL AND INTERCARPAL JOINTS)

Type of joint: This joint is classified as a condyloid joint with two degrees of freedom (flexion and extension, radial and ulnar deviation). The articulation of the proximal and distal rows of metacarpals are of the same classification and also allow for flexion and extension.

Capsular pattern: Equal restriction of all motions.

Wrist Flexion

Planes/axis of movement: Motion occurs in the sagittal plane around a coronal axis primarily at the radiocarpal joint. Flexion also occurs at the midcarpal joint to a lesser degree, while the proximal row of carpal bones glide posteriorly on the distal end of the radius.

Range of motion:

- 0 degrees to 50 degrees (at the radiocarpal joint)
- 0 degrees to 35 degrees (at the midcarpal joint)
- 0 degrees to 90 degrees (from the anatomical position)

Preferred starting position: See Figure 2-43.

End position: See Figure 2-44.

Goniometric alignment:

- Axis: Center over the lateral aspect of the wrist, just distal to the styloid process of the ulna
- Stationary arm: Align with the lateral midline of the ulna, siting the olecranon process
- Moving arm: Align with the lateral midline of the fifth metacarpal bone

Stabilization: The forearm should be stabilized on a supporting surface.

Substitutions: The examiner must watch to make sure the forearm stays down on the table and the wrist does not drift into ulnar/radial deviation to avoid pain or gain more flexion.

Alternate method/position for testing: See Figure 2-45.

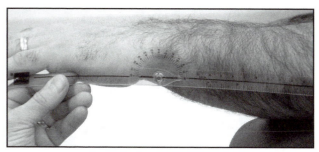

Figure 2-43. The subject should be sitting with the forearm resting on a table with the palm facing down. The shoulder should be abducted to 90 degrees with the elbow flexed to 90 degrees; the fingers should be loosely in extension.

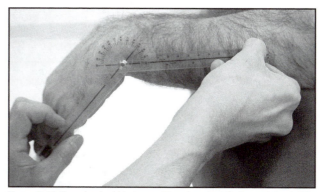

Figure 2-44. The wrist should be in a position of maximal flexion at the end of the movement.

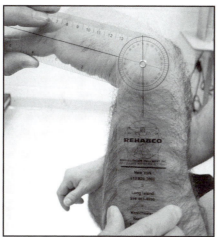

Figure 2-45. The subject is sitting with the elbow flexed to 90 degrees with the olecranon process sitting on the table surface. The forearm is placed in a neutral position between pronation and supination. The fingers are held loosely in flexion.

Wrist Extension/Hyperextension

Planes/axis of movement: Motion occurs in the sagittal plane around a coronal axis at both the radiocarpal and midcarpal joint, with extension occurring more extensively at the latter.

Range of motion:

- 90 degrees to 0 degrees (from full flexion)
- 0 degrees to 70 degrees (hyperextension)

Preferred starting position: See Figure 2-46.

End position: See Figure 2-47.

Goniometric alignment:

- Axis: At the lateral aspect of the wrist, just distal to the ulnar styloid
- Stationary arm: Align with the lateral midline of the ulna, siting the olecranon process
- Moving arm: Align with the lateral midline of the fifth metacarpal bone

Stabilization: The forearm should be stabilized against a supporting surface.

Substitutions: The examiner should watch to make sure the forearm does not rise off the table or the wrist does not drift into ulnar/radial deviation to avoid a painful movement or to gain more extension.

Alternate method/position for testing: See Figure 2-48.

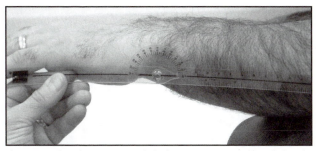

Figure 2-46. The subject is sitting with the forearm resting on a table with the palm facing down. The shoulder and elbow should be flexed to 90 degrees and the fingers should be held loosely in flexion.

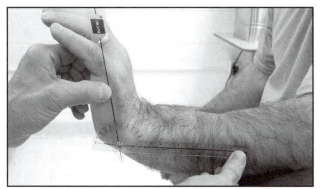

Figure 2-47. The wrist should be in a position of maximal extension/hyperextension at the end of the movement.

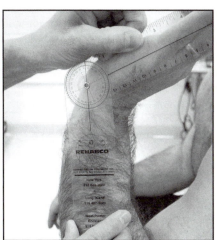

Figure 2-48. The subject is sitting with the elbow flexed to 90 degrees with the olecranon process sitting on the table surface. The forearm is placed in a neutral position between pronation and supination. The fingers are held in extension.

Wrist Radial Deviation (Abduction)

Planes/axis of movement: Motion occurs in the frontal/coronal plane in the anatomic position around an anterior/posterior axis. In the testing position, motion occurs in the transverse plane around a vertical axis. The motion occurs between the radiocarpal joint and the intercarpal bones.

Range of motion:

- 0 degrees to 25 degrees

Preferred starting position: See Figure 2-49.

End position: See Figure 2-50.

Goniometric alignment:

- Axis: Align over the middle of the dorsal surface of the wrist, over the capitate

- Stationary arm: Align with the dorsal midline of the forearm, siting the lateral epicondyle of the humerus

- Moving arm: Align with the midline of the dorsal surface of the third metacarpal

Stabilization: The distal ends of the radius and ulna must be stabilized against a supporting surface.

Substitutions: The subject may try to flex or extend the wrist or move the forearm into supination or pronation to avoid pain or gain more radial deviation.

Alternate method/position for testing: The subject may lie in supine if necessary with the palm facing down on the table.

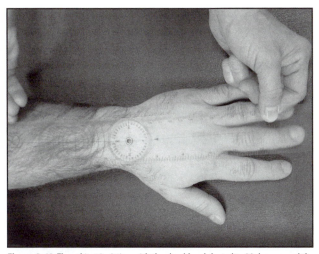

Figure 2-49. The subject is sitting with the shoulder abducted to 90 degrees and the elbow flexed to 90 degrees. The forearm rests on a supporting surface with the palm down. The wrist should be neutrally positioned between radial and ulnar deviation.

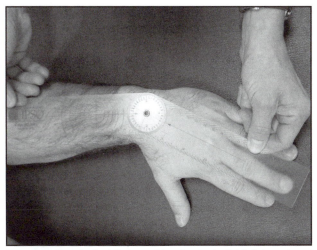

Figure 2-50. The wrist should be in a position of maximal radial deviation at the end of the movement.

Wrist Ulnar Deviation (Adduction)

Planes/axis of movement: Motion occurs in the frontal/coronal plane in the anatomic position around an anterior/posterior axis. In the testing position, motion occurs in the transverse plane around a vertical axis. The motion occurs between the radiocarpal joint and the intercarpal bones.

Range of motion:

- 0 degrees to 35 degrees

Preferred starting position: See Figure 2-51.

End position: See Figure 2-52.

Goniometric alignment:

- Axis: Align the axis over the middle of the dorsal aspect of the wrist over the capitate

- Stationary arm: Align with the dorsal midline of the forearm, siting the lateral epicondyle of the humerus

- Moving arm: Align with the midline of the dorsal surface of the third metacarpal

Stabilization: The distal ends of the radius and ulna must be stabilized against a supporting surface.

Substitutions: The subject may try to flex or extend the wrist or move the forearm into supination or pronation to avoid pain or gain more ulnar deviation.

Alternate method/position for testing: The subject may lie in supine if necessary with the palm facing down on the table.

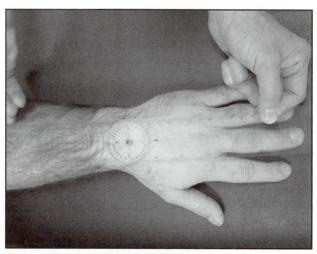

Figure 2-51. The subject is sitting with the shoulder abducted to 90 degrees and the elbow flexed to 90 degrees. The forearm rests on a supporting surface with the palm down. The wrist should be neutrally positioned between radial and ulnar deviation.

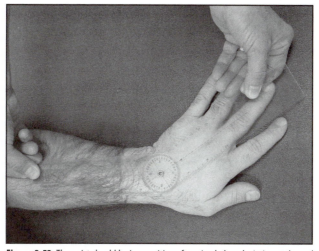

Figure 2-52. The wrist should be in a position of maximal ulnar deviation at the end of the movement.

THE FINGERS—DIGITS II TO V (METACARPOPHALANGEAL JOINTS)

Type of joint: Condyloid, with the convex surfaces of the heads of the metacarpals articulating with the concave surfaces of the proximal phalanges.

Capsular pattern: Flexion > extension.

MCP Flexion

Planes/axis of movement: Motion occurs in the sagittal plane around a transverse axis in the anatomical position, but in the testing position, motion occurs in the transverse plane around a vertical axis. Motion occurs between individual metacarpals and the corresponding phalanx, with the phalanx moving anteriorly on the metacarpal.

Range of motion:

- 0 degrees to 90 degrees of flexion (when moving with full extension of the interphalangeal joints)

Preferred starting position: See Figure 2-53.

End position: See Figure 2-54.

Goniometric alignment:

- Axis: Over the dorsal aspect of the MCP joint
- Stationary arm: Align over the dorsal midline of the metacarpal bone
- Moving arm: Align over the dorsal midline of the proximal phalanx

Stabilization: The tested metacarpal must be stabilized to prevent wrist motion.

Substitutions: The subject may try to flex or deviate the wrist to avoid the movement because of pain.

Alternate method/position for testing: The subject may lie supine with the forearm lying in a neutral position on a supporting surface and with the wrist and fingers in a neutral position.

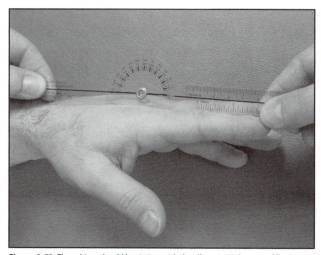

Figure 2-53. The subject should be sitting with the elbow in 90 degrees of flexion and the forearm should be in a neutral position between supination and pronation. The wrist and fingers should be in a neutral position.

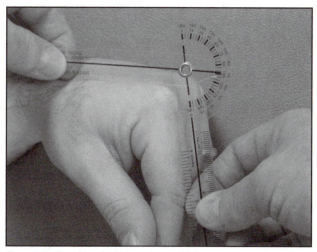

Figure 2-54. The subject should move the tested MCP joint into maximal flexion.

MCP Extension/Hyperextension

Planes/axis of movement: Movement occurs in a transverse plane around a vertical axis when testing. Motion is considered hyperextension when it occurs beyond 0 degrees of extension.

Range of motion:

- 90 degrees to 0 degrees (extension)
- 0 degrees to 30 degrees (hyperextension)

Preferred starting position: See Figure 2-55.

End position: See Figure 2-56.

Goniometric alignment:

- Axis: Over the dorsal aspect of the MCP joint
- Stationary arm: Align over the dorsal midline of the metacarpal bone
- Moving arm: Align over the dorsal midline of the proximal phalanx

Stabilization: The tested metacarpal must be stabilized to prevent wrist motion.

Substitutions: The subject may try to deviate the wrist to avoid movement because of pain.

Alternate method/position for testing: See Figure 2-57.

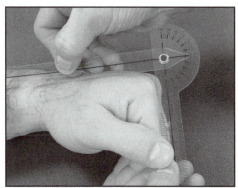

Figure 2-55. The subject should be sitting with the elbow in 90 degrees of flexion, with the forearm and wrist in neutral, and with the MCP joints in full flexion.

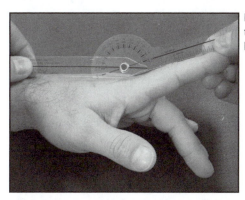

Figure 2-56. The subject should move the tested MCP joint into maximal extension/ hyperextension.

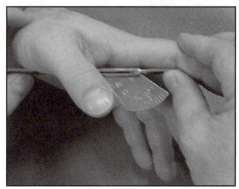

Figure 2-57. The goniometer may be placed on the palmar surface of the MCP joint to measure hyperextension.

MCP Abduction

Planes/axis of movement: Motion occurs in the frontal plane around an anterior/posterior plane in the anatomical position. Motion occurs in the transverse plane around a vertical axis during testing. The second digit moves radially from the third digit, and the fourth and fifth digits move ulnarly from the middle finger.

Range of motion:

- 0 degrees to 20 degrees

Preferred starting position: See Figure 2-58.

End position: See Figure 2-59.

Goniometric alignment:

- Axis: Over the dorsal aspect of the MCP joint
- Stationary arm: Align over the dorsal midline of the metacarpal bone
- Moving arm: Align over the dorsal aspect of the proximal phalanx

Stabilization: The tested metacarpal must be stabilized to prevent wrist movement.

Substitutions: The subject may try to deviate the wrist into radial or ulnar deviation or into extension to avoid pain or gain motion with testing.

Alternate method/position for testing: The subject may lie supine with the elbow extended and the forearm lying in neutral on a supporting surface and with the wrist and fingers in neutral.

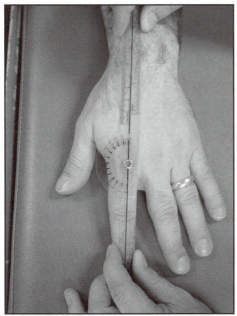

Figure 2-58. The subject should be sitting with the elbow flexed to 90 degrees and with the forearm in pronation with the palm facing the floor. The wrist should be in a neutral position between radial and ulnar deviation and the fingers should be extended.

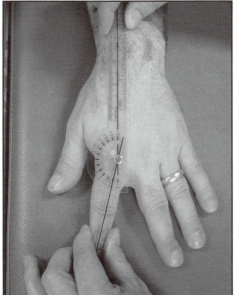

Figure 2-59. The subject should move the tested metacarpal into a position of maximal MCP abduction.

MCP Adduction

Planes/axis of movement: This is the return motion from MCP abduction. Motion occurs in the transverse plane around a vertical axis. The second digit moves in an ulnar direction, while the fourth and fifth digits move radially toward the middle finger.

Range of motion:

- 0 degrees to 20 degrees (with the middle finger positioned to allow for 20 degrees of motion to occur from the anatomical position)

Preferred starting position: See Figure 2-60.

End position: See Figure 2-61.

Goniometric alignment:

- Axis: Position over the dorsal aspect of the MCP joint
- Stationary arm: Align over the dorsal midline of the metacarpal bone
- Moving arm: Align over the dorsal aspect of the proximal phalanx

Stabilization: The tested metacarpal must be stabilized to prevent wrist movement.

Substitutions: The subject may try to deviate, flex, or extend the wrist to gain more movement or flex the MCP joints to gain more movement with testing.

Alternate method/position for testing: The subject may lie in supine with the elbow extended and with the forearm lying in neutral on a supporting surface, with the wrist and fingers in neutral.

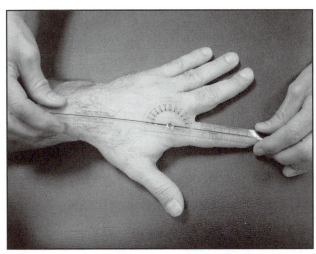

Figure 2-60. The subject should be sitting with the elbow flexed to 90 degrees and with the forearm in pronation with the palm facing the floor. The wrist should be in a neutral position between radial and ulnar deviation and the fingers should be extended.

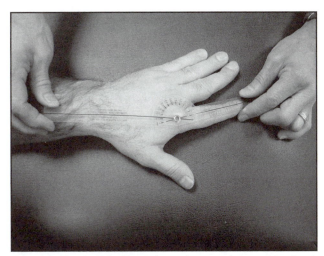

Figure 2-61. The subject should move the tested metacarpal into a position of maximal MCP adduction.

THE FINGERS—DIGITS II TO V (PROXIMAL INTERPHALANGEAL JOINTS)

Type of joint: Hinge joint with one degree of freedom, allowing only for flexion and extension.

Capsular pattern: Flexion > extension.

PIP Flexion

Planes/axis of movement: In the testing position, movement occurs in the transverse plane around a vertical axis.

Range of motion:

- 0 degrees to 120 degrees

Preferred starting position: See Figure 2-62.

End position: See Figure 2-63.

Goniometric alignment:

- Axis: Over the dorsal aspect of the PIP joint

- Stationary arm: Align over the dorsal midline of the proximal phalanx

- Moving arm: Align over the dorsal midline of the middle phalanx

Stabilization: The proximal phalanx should be stabilized to prevent motion at the MCP joint or wrist.

Substitutions: The subject may try to flex the wrist or MCP joint to avoid pain with the movement.

Alternate method/position for testing: None.

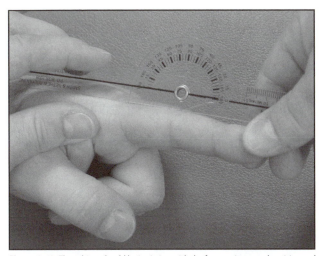

Figure 2-62. The subject should be in sitting with the forearm in neutral position and with the wrist and hand supported on a tabletop. The MCP, PIP, and DIP joints should be in a neutral position.

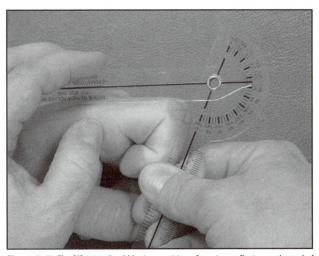

Figure 2-63. The PIP joint should be in a position of maximum flexion at the end of the movement.

PIP Extension

Planes/axis of movement: In the testing position, motion occurs in the transverse plane around a vertical axis.

Range of motion:

- 120 degrees to 0 degrees (from full flexion)
- 0 degrees to 10 degrees (hyperextension)

Preferred starting position: See Figure 2-64.

End position: See Figure 2-65.

Goniometric alignment:

- Axis: Over the dorsal aspect of the PIP joint
- Stationary arm: Align over the midline of the dorsal aspect of the proximal phalanx
- Moving arm: Align over the midline of the dorsal aspect of the middle phalanx

Stabilization: The proximal phalanx should be stabilized to prevent motion at the MCP joint or wrist.

Substitutions: The subject may try to extend the MCP joint or wrist to avoid pain or gain more movement during testing.

Alternate method/position for testing: See Figure 2-66.

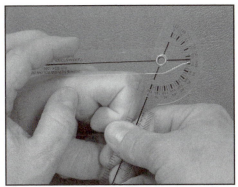

Figure 2-64. The subject should be in sitting with the forearm in neutral position and with the wrist and hand supported on a tabletop. The PIP and DIP joints should be in full flexion.

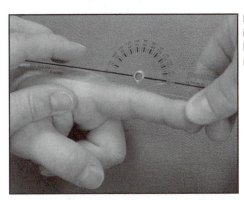

Figure 2-65. The PIP joint should be in a position of maximum extension/hyperextension at the end of the movement.

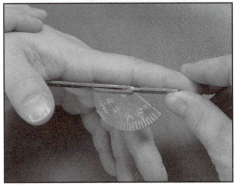

Figure 2-66. The goniometer may be placed on the palmar surface of the PIP joint to measure hyperextension.

THE FINGERS—DIGITS II TO V (DISTAL INTERPHALANGEAL JOINTS)

Type of joint: Hinge joint with one degree of freedom allowing only for flexion and extension.

Capsular pattern: Flexion > extension.

DIP Flexion

Planes/axis of movement: In the testing position, motion occurs in the transverse plane around a vertical axis.

Range of motion:

■ 0 degrees to 80 degrees

Preferred starting position: See Figure 2-67.

End position: See Figure 2-68.

Goniometric alignment:

■ Axis: Over the dorsal aspect of the DIP joint

■ Stationary arm: Align over the dorsal midline of the middle phalanx

■ Moving arm: Align over the dorsal midline of the distal phalanx

Stabilization: The middle phalanx of the tested digit should be stabilized to prevent further flexion of the PIP and MCP joints.

Substitutions: The subject may try to slightly raise the forearm to avoid pain with movement.

Alternate method/position for testing: None.

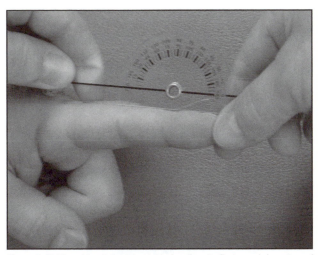

Figure 2-67. The subject is in sitting with the elbow in flexion and the wrist and fingers in a neutral position, resting on a tabletop.

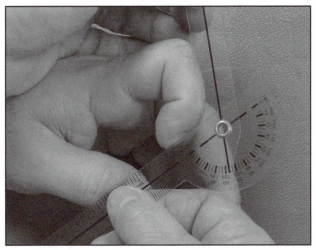

Figure 2-68. The DIP joint should be in a position of maximal flexion at the end of the movement.

DIP Extension

Planes/axis of movement: In the testing position, motion occurs in a transverse plane around a vertical axis.

Range of motion:

- 80 degrees to 0 degrees (extension)
- 0 degrees to 10 degrees (hyperextension)

Preferred starting position: See Figure 2-69.

End position: See Figure 2-70.

Goniometric alignment:

- Axis: Over the dorsal aspect of the DIP joint
- Stationary arm: Align with the dorsal midline of the middle phalanx
- Moving arm: Align with the dorsal midline of the distal phalanx

Stabilization: The middle phalanx should be stabilized to prevent excessive extension of the PIP and MCP joints.

Substitutions: The subject may try to extend the PIP joint, MCP joint, or wrist to avoid pain with movement.

Alternate method/position for testing: See Figure 2-71.

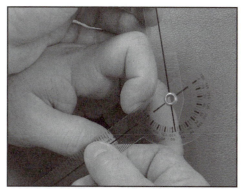

Figure 2-69. The subject should be in sitting with the elbow flexed and the forearm and wrist in a neutral position resting on a tabletop. The PIP joint is flexed to approximately 80 degrees and the DIP joint should be in maximum flexion.

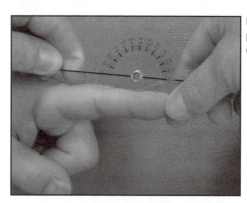

Figure 2-70. The DIP joint should be in a position of maximum extension at the end of the movement.

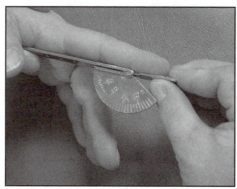

Figure 2-71. The goniometer may be placed on the palmar surface of the DIP joint to measure hyperextension.

THE THUMB (CARPOMETACARPAL JOINT)

Type of joint: A saddle joint with multiple degrees of freedom, allowing for opposition and reposition of the thumb to occur.

Capsular pattern: Abduction > extension.

CMC Flexion

Planes/axis of movement: Movement occurs in the frontal plane around an anterior/posterior axis in the anatomic position. In the testing position, movement occurs in the transverse plane around a vertical axis.

Range of motion:

- 0 degrees to 15 degrees

Preferred starting position: See Figure 2-72.

End position: See Figure 2-73.

Goniometric alignment:

- Axis: Center over the palmar aspect of the CMC joint

- Stationary arm: Align over the palmar midline of the radial shaft

- Moving arm: Align over the palmar midline of the first metacarpal bone

> The goniometer arms may not align at 0 degrees in the start position, although the start position is recorded as such (ie, the start position may read 30 degrees). The range of motion for this movement is recorded as the total number of degrees between the start position and end position. Therefore, a measurement that begins with 30 degrees and ends at 15 degrees should be recorded as 0 to 15 degrees.

Stabilization: The forearm and wrist should be stabilized against a supporting surface to prevent wrist movement.

Substitutions: The subject may try to attempt to flex or ulnarly deviate the wrist to avoid the movement because of pain or to gain more motion. The examiner must also watch that the thumb does not move into opposition.

Alternate method/position for testing: None.

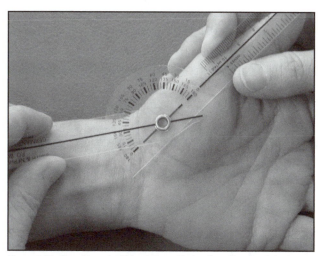

Figure 2-72. The subject should be sitting with the elbow flexed and the forearm in supination. The forearm and hand should rest on a tabletop. The wrist and MCP and IP joints of the thumb should be in a neutral position. The CMC joint should be in midposition between abduction and adduction.

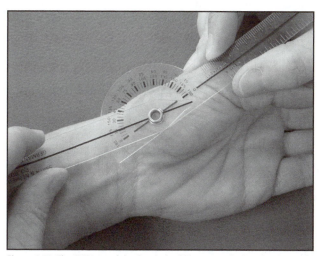

Figure 2-73. The CMC joint of the thumb should be maximally flexed at the end of the motion.

CMC Extension

Planes/axis of movement: Movement occurs in the frontal plane around an anterior/posterior axis in the anatomic position. In the testing position, movement occurs in the transverse plane around a vertical axis.

Range of motion:

- 0 degrees to 20 degrees

Preferred starting position: See Figure 2-74.

End position: See Figure 2-75.

Goniometric alignment:

- Axis: Center over the palmar aspect of the CMC joint

- Stationary arm: Align over the palmar midline of the radius

- Moving arm: Align over the palmar midline of the first metacarpal bone

> The goniometer arms may not align at 0 degrees in the start position, although the start position is recorded as such (ie, the start position may read 30 degrees). The range of motion for this movement is recorded as the total number of degrees between the start and end position. Therefore, a measurement that begins with 30 degrees and ends at 50 degrees should be recorded as 0 to 20 degrees.

Stabilization: The forearm and wrist must be stabilized against a supporting surface to prevent wrist movement.

Substitutions: The subject may try to extend or radially deviate the wrist to increase the motion or avoid pain. The subject may also abduct the thumb to avoid pain.

Alternate method/position for testing: None.

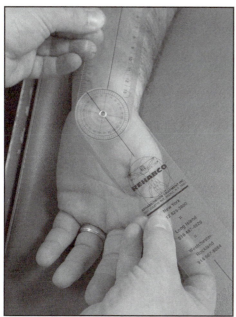

Figure 2-74. The subject should be sitting with the elbow flexed and the forearm in supination. The forearm and hand should rest on a tabletop. The wrist and MCP and IP joints of the thumb should be in a neutral position. The CMC joint should be in midposition between abduction and adduction.

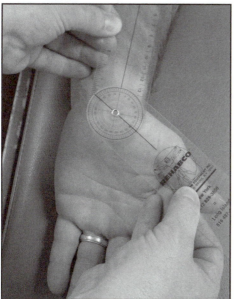

Figure 2-75. The CMC joint of the thumb should be maximally extended at the end of the movement.

CMC Abduction

Planes/axis of movement: During testing, motion occurs in a transverse plane around a vertical axis. The thumb moves at a right angle to the palm.

Range of motion:

■ 0 degrees to 60 degrees

Preferred starting position: See Figure 2-76.

End position: See Figure 2-77.

Goniometric alignment:

■ Axis: Center over the dorsal aspect of the CMC joint

■ Stationary arm: Align with the lateral midline of the second metacarpal bone

■ Moving arm: Align with the lateral midline of the first metacarpal bone

---

The goniometer arms may not align at 0 degrees in the start position, although the start position is recorded as such (ie, the start position may read 15 to 20 degrees). The range of motion for this movement is recorded as the total number of degrees between the start and end position. Therefore, a measurement that begins at 15 degrees and ends at 60 degrees should be recorded as 45 degrees of CMC abduction.

Stabilization: The wrist and second metacarpal should be stabilized against a supporting surface to prevent wrist movement.

Substitutions: The subject may try to flex or extend the wrist or oppose the thumb to increase movement or to avoid pain during testing.

Alternate method/position for testing: None.

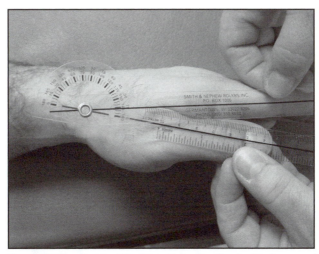

Figure 2-76. The subject should be sitting with the elbow flexed and the forearm and wrist in a neutral position resting on a tabletop. The CMC, MCP, and IP joints should be in a neutral position between flexion and extension.

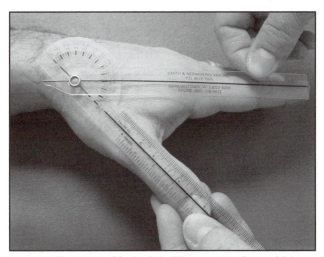

Figure 2-77. The CMC joint of the thumb should be in a position of maximal abduction at the end of the movement.

CMC Adduction

Planes/axis of movement: During testing, motion occurs in a transverse plane around a vertical axis.

Range of motion:

- 60 degrees to 0 degrees

Preferred starting position: See Figure 2-78.

End position: See Figure 2-79.

Goniometric alignment:

- Axis: Center over the dorsal aspect of the CMC joint
- Stationary arm: Align with the lateral midline of the second metacarpal bone
- Moving arm: Align with the lateral midline of the first metacarpal bone

---

The goniometer arms will not align at 0 degrees at the start position, although the start position is recorded as such (ie, the start position may read 60 degrees). The range of motion for this movement is recorded as the total number of degrees between the start and end position. Therefore, a measurement that begins at 60 degrees and ends at 15 degrees should be recorded as 45 degrees of CMC adduction.

Stabilization: The wrist and second metacarpal should be stabilized against a supporting surface to prevent wrist movement.

Substitutions: The subject may try to flex, extend, or oppose the thumb to increase movement or to avoid pain during testing.

Alternate method/position for testing: None.

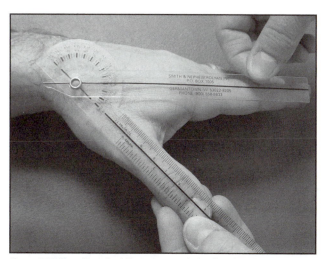

Figure 2-78. The subject should be in sitting with the elbow flexed and the forearm and wrist in a neutral position resting on a tabletop. The CMC should be in full abduction and the MCP and IP joints should be in a neutral position between flexion and extension.

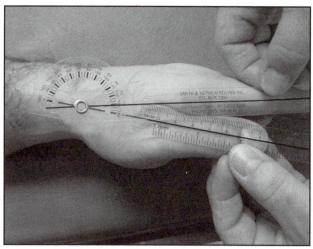

Figure 2-79. The CMC joint of the thumb should be in a position of maximal adduction at the end of the movement.

CMC Opposition

Planes/axis of movement: This motion combines the movements of flexion, abduction, and internal rotation of the first metacarpal and trapezium. The thumb moves toward the tip of the fifth digit with the pad of the thumb touching the pad of the fifth digit. It moves through a varying array of planes and axes.

Range of motion:

- Variable, "normal" range of motion allows for complete motion until the tips of the thumb and fifth digit meet from an open-palm position

Preferred starting position: See Figure 2-80.

End position: See Figure 2-81.

Goniometric alignment:

- In this motion, a ruler is used in place of a goniometer to record the deficit of complete range of motion. The ruler is placed from the tip of the thumb to the tip of the fifth digit.

Stabilization: The fifth metacarpal should be stabilized against a supporting surface to prevent wrist movement.

Substitutions: The subject may try to attempt to flex the wrist to increase the motion.

Alternate method/position for testing: None.

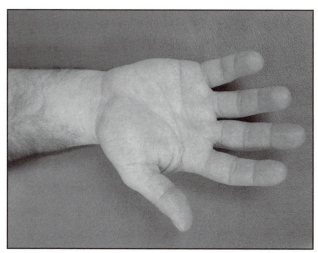

Figure 2-80. The subject is sitting with the elbow flexed and the forearm supported in a fully supinated position. The wrist is in a neutral position and the IP joint of the thumb and fifth digit are in a neutral position between flexion and extension.

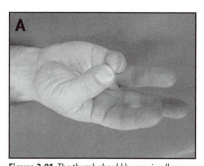

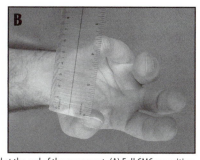

Figure 2-81. The thumb should be maximally opposed at the end of the movement. (A) Full CMC opposition. (B) CMC opposition deficit.

THE THUMB
(METACARPOPHALANGEAL JOINT)

Type of joint: Hinge joint that allows for one degree of freedom in flexion and extension.

Capsular pattern: Flexion > extension.

MCP Flexion

Planes/axis of movement: Movement occurs in the transverse plane around a vertical axis during testing.

Range of motion:

■ 0 degrees to 50 degrees

Preferred starting position: See Figure 2-82.

End position: See Figure 2-83.

Goniometric alignment:

■ Axis: Center over the dorsal aspect of the MCP joint

■ Stationary arm: Align over the dorsal midline of the first metacarpal bone

■ Moving arm: Align over the dorsal midline of the proximal phalanx

Stabilization: The first metacarpal and CMC joint of the thumb should be stabilized.

Substitutions: The subject may try to flex the wrist to increase the movement or avoid pain during testing.

Alternate method/position for testing: None.

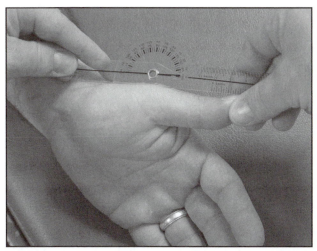

Figure 2-82. The subject is in sitting with the elbow flexed. The forearm should be in supination with the wrist in a neutral position. The CMC and IP joints should be in a neutral position. The forearm, wrist, and hand should be resting on a tabletop.

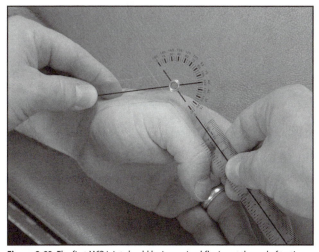

Figure 2-83. The first MCP joint should be in maximal flexion at the end of testing.

MCP Extension/Hyperextension

Planes/axis of movement: This motion is the return movement from thumb MCP flexion. This movement occurs in the transverse plane around a vertical axis during testing.

Range of motion:

- 50 degrees to 0 degrees (extension)
- 0 degrees to 10 degrees (hyperextension)

Preferred starting position: See Figure 2-84.

End position: See Figure 2-85.

Goniometric alignment:

- Axis: Center over the dorsal surface of the MCP joint
- Stationary arm: Align along the dorsal surface of the first metacarpal bone
- Moving arm: Align along the dorsal midline of the proximal phalanx of the thumb

Stabilization: The first metacarpal and CMC joint of the thumb should be stabilized.

Substitutions: The subject may try to flex or radially deviate the wrist to gain more motion or avoid pain during movement.

Alternate method/position for testing: See Figure 2-86.

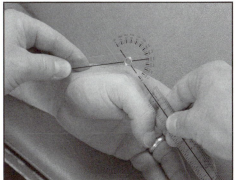

Figure 2-84. The subject is sitting with the elbow flexed, the forearm in supination, and with the wrist and fingers in a neutral position. The first MCP joint should be in full flexion. The forearm, wrist, and hand should be resting on a tabletop.

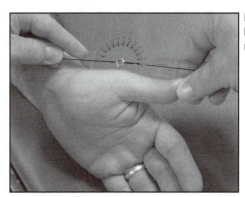

Figure 2-85. The first MCP joint should be in maximal extension at the end of the movement.

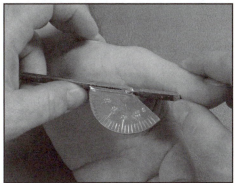

Figure 2-86. The goniometer may be placed on the palmar surface of the MCP joint to measure hyperextension.

THE THUMB (INTERPHALANGEAL JOINT)

Type of joint: Hinge joint with one degree of freedom allowing only for flexion and extension.

Capsular pattern: Flexion > extension.

IP Flexion

Planes/axis of movement: Movement occurs in the transverse plane around a vertical axis during testing.

Range of motion:

- 0 degrees to 90 degrees

Preferred starting position: See Figure 2-87.

End position: See Figure 2-88.

Goniometric alignment:

- Axis: Center over the dorsal surface of the IP joint
- Stationary arm: Align with the dorsal midline of the proximal phalanx
- Moving arm: Align with the dorsal midline of the distal phalanx

Stabilization: The proximal phalanx of the thumb should be stabilized.

Substitutions: The subject may try to flex the wrist or first MCP joint to increase the amount of the range of motion or avoid pain during testing.

Alternate method/position for testing: None.

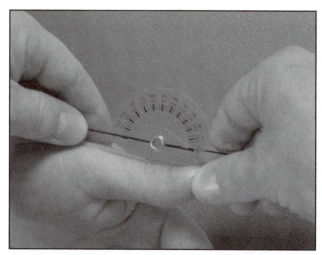

Figure 2-87. The subject is sitting with the elbow flexed and the forearm in full supination. The wrist and CMC joints of the thumb should be in a neutral position. The forearm and hand should rest on a tabletop.

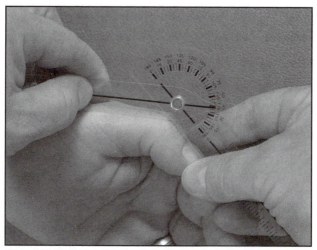

Figure 2-88. The IP joint of the thumb should be maximally flexed at the end of the movement.

IP Extension/Hyperextension

Planes/axis of movement: Movement occurs in the transverse plane around a vertical axis during testing. This is the return motion from full thumb IP flexion.

Range of motion:

- 90 degrees to 0 degrees

Preferred starting position: See Figure 2-89.

End position: See Figure 2-90.

Goniometric alignment:

- Axis: Center over the dorsal aspect of the IP joint
- Stationary arm: Align over the dorsal midline of the proximal phalanx
- Moving arm: Align over the dorsal midline of the distal phalanx

Stabilization: The proximal phalanx of the thumb should be stabilized.

Substitutions: The subject may try to extend the wrist, CMC joint, or first MCP joint to increase the range of motion during testing.

Alternate method/position for testing: See Figure 2-91.

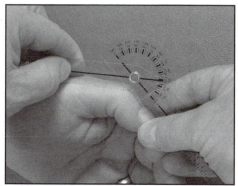

Figure 2-89. The subject is in sitting with the elbow flexed and the forearm fully supinated. The wrist, CMC joint, and MCP joint of the thumb should be in a neutral position with the IP joint in full flexion.

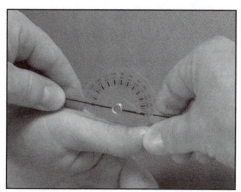

Figure 2-90. The IP joint of the thumb should be in maximal extension at the end of the movement.

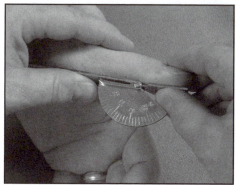

Figure 2-91. The goniometer may be placed on the palmar surface of the IP joint to measure hyperextension.

SECTION III

Thoracic and Lumbar Spine

L. Van Ost
Cram Session in Goniometry:
A Handbook for Students & Clinicians (pp. 87-95)
© 2010 SLACK Incorporated

THE THORACOLUMBAR SPINE

Type of joint: The thoracic and lumbar spine are very complex structures involving segmented movement at numerous vertebral articulations. As a result, it is not possible to accurately measure all movements occurring along this area of the spine with a goniometer. An alternative method will be addressed.

Capsular pattern: Lateral flexion = rotation/extension.

Thoracolumbar Flexion

Planes/axis of movement: Movement occurs in the sagittal plane around a coronal axis.

Range of motion:

- Approximately 4-inch difference between initial and ending measurements

Preferred starting position: See Figure 3-1.

End position: See Figure 3-2.

Measurement of motion: The distance between the spinous processes of C7 and S1 is first measured in standing. The subject then flexes the trunk as far forward as possible and the second measurement is taken. The difference between the two measurements is the amount of flexion present.

Stabilization: The pelvis should be stabilized to prevent anterior tilting. Stabilization is achieved through subject compliance.

Substitutions: See Figure 3-3.

Alternate method/position for testing: None.

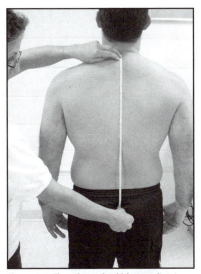

Figure 3-1. The subject should be standing in an erect position with the arms by the sides.

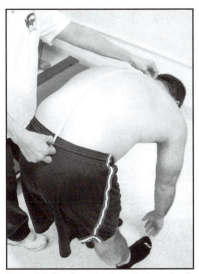

Figure 3-2. The thoracolumbar spine is maximally flexed forward.

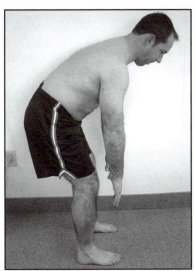

Figure 3-3. The subject may try to flex the hips and/or the knees during movement to gain more flexion. This may occur as the hamstrings are maximally stretched.

Thoracolumbar Extension/Hyperextension

Planes/axis of movement: Extension is the return motion from full thoracolumbar flexion. Beyond 0 degrees starting position is considered hyperextension. Motion occurs in the sagittal plane around a coronal axis.

Range of motion:

- Approximately 2-inch difference between the initial and ending measurements

Preferred starting position: See Figure 3-4.

End position: See Figure 3-5.

Measurement of motion: The distance between the spinous processes of C7 and S1 is first measured in standing. The subject extends the trunk as far backward as possible and a second measurement is taken. The difference between the two measurements is the amount of extension present.

Stabilization: The pelvis should be stabilized to prevent posterior tilting. Stabilization is achieved through subject compliance.

Substitutions: See Figure 3-6.

Alternate method/position for testing: None.

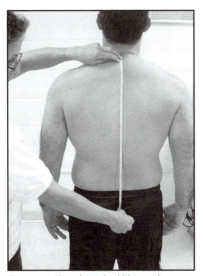

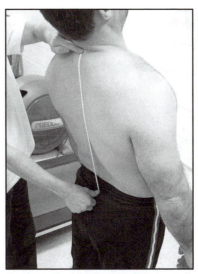

Figure 3-4. The subject should be standing in an erect position with the arms by the sides.

Figure 3-5. The thoracolumbar spine is maximally extended at the end of the motion.

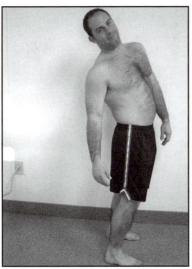

Figure 3-6. The subject may try to laterally bend or rotate the trunk during testing to gain more motion or avoid pain. The subject may also bend the knees as the hip flexors are maximally stretched.

Thoracolumbar Lateral Flexion

Planes/axis of movement: Motion occurs in the frontal plane around an anterior/posterior axis.

Range of motion:

- Range of motion is variable because of the differences in arm and trunk length. The amount of motion is determined by the comparison of both sides.

Preferred starting position: See Figure 3-7.

End position: See Figure 3-8.

Measurement of motion: The distance between the tip of the middle finger and floor is taken first. The subject then laterally flexes to the side as far as possible and a second measurement is taken. The difference between the two measurements is the amount of lateral flexion present.

Stabilization: The pelvis should be stabilized during testing. Stabilization is achieved through subject compliance.

Substitutions: See Figure 3-9.

Alternate method/position for testing: None.

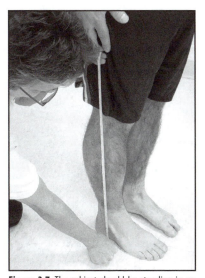

Figure 3-7. The subject should be standing in an erect position with the arms by the sides.

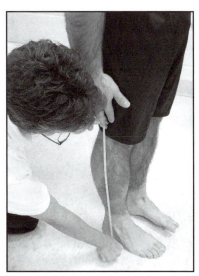

Figure 3-8. The thoracolumbar spine is maximally laterally flexed to the tested side.

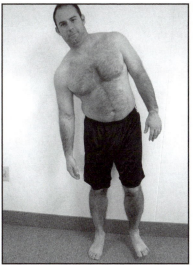

Figure 3-9. The subject may try to flex, extend, or rotate the trunk during testing or lift the opposite lower extremity off the floor to gain more motion.

Thoracolumbar Rotation

Planes/axis of movement: Motion occurs in the transverse plane around a vertical axis.

Range of motion:

■ 0 degrees to 45 degrees

Preferred starting position: See Figure 3-10.

End position: See Figure 3-11.

Goniometric alignment:

■ Axis: Align over the center of the top of the head

■ Stationary arm: Align parallel to an imaginary line between the two iliac crests

■ Moving arm: Align parallel to the top of the shoulder, siting the acromion process

Stabilization: The pelvis should be stabilized during testing. Stabilization is achieved through subject compliance.

Substitutions: The subject may try to flex, extend, or laterally flex the trunk to increase the motion. He/she may also try to raise the pelvis.

Alternate method/position for testing: None.

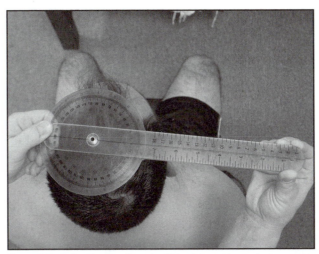

Figure 3-10. Preferably, the subject should be sitting without a back support to ensure full mobility. The cervical, thoracic, and lumbar spine should be in a neutral position with the arms resting by the sides.

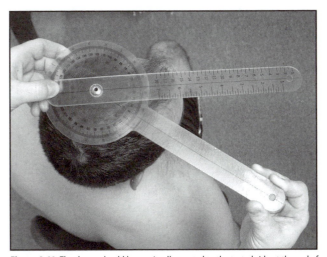

Figure 3-11. The thorax should be maximally rotated to the tested side at the end of the movement.

SECTION IV

Lower Extremity

L. Van Ost
Cram Session in Goniometry:
A Handbook for Students & Clinicians (pp. 97-149)
© 2010 SLACK Incorporated

THE HIP

Type of joint: Ball and socket joint with three degrees of freedom.

Capsular pattern: Internal/external rotation > abduction > flexion > extension > adduction.

Hip Flexion

Planes/axis of movement: Motion occurs in the sagittal plane around a coronal axis. During testing, the knee is allowed to flex passively so the hamstrings do not limit movement.

Range of motion:

- 0 degrees to 115 (with the knee extended)
- 0 degrees to 125 (with the knee flexed)

Preferred starting position: See Figure 4-1.

End position: See Figure 4-2.

Goniometric alignment:

- Axis: Center on the lateral aspect of the hip joint over the greater trochanter of the femur
- Stationary arm: Align parallel to the lateral midline of the trunk
- Moving arm: Align parallel to the lateral midline of the femur, siting the lateral epicondyle

Stabilization: The pelvis should be stabilized against a supporting surface by the weight of the body.

Substitutions: The subject may try to flex the lumbar spine or opposite hip during testing.

Alternate method/position for testing: See Figure 4-3.

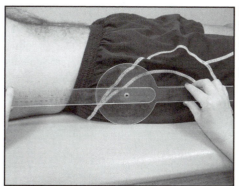

Figure 4-1. The subject lies supine with the hip in midposition between abduction, adduction, and rotation. The opposite lower extremity is extended and rests on a supporting surface.

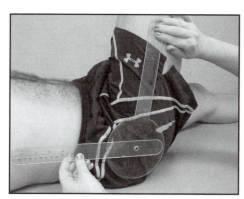

Figure 4-2. The hip should be in a position of maximum hip flexion at the end of the movement.

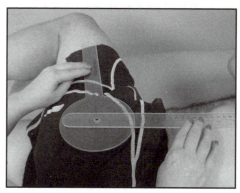

Figure 4-3. The subject may be positioned in sidelying on the uninvolved side.

Hip Extension/Hyperextension

Planes/axis of movement: Movement occurs in the sagittal plane around a coronal axis. Extension and hyperextension are the "return" movements from a position of hip flexion.

Range of motion:

■ 125 degrees to 0 degrees (extension)

■ 0 degrees to 15 degrees (hyperextension)

Preferred starting position: See Figure 4-4.

End position: See Figure 4-5.

Goniometric alignment

■ Axis: Center on the lateral aspect of the hip joint over the greater trochanter of the femur

■ Stationary arm: Align parallel to the lateral midline of the trunk

■ Moving arm: Align parallel to the lateral midline of the femur, siting the lateral epicondyle

Stabilization: The pelvis should be stabilized against a supporting surface by the weight of the body, a strap, or the clinician's hand if necessary.

Substitutions: The subject may try to extend the lumbar spine or rotate the hips to avoid pain or increase the motion.

Alternate method/position for testing: The subject may be positioned in sidelying on the uninvolved side. The nontested hip should be flexed to 90 degrees to prevent anterior pelvic tilting.

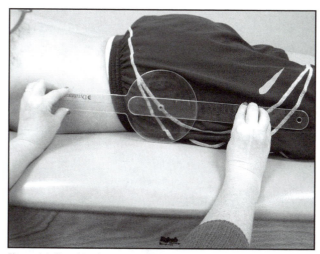

Figure 4-4. The subject lies prone with the lower extremities in full extension with both hips in a neutral position.

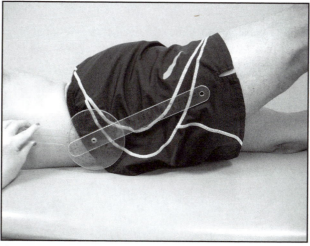

Figure 4-5. The hip should be in a position of maximal hip extension at the end of the movement.

Hip Abduction

Planes/axis of movement: Movement occurs in a frontal plane around an anterior/posterior axis.

Range of motion:

- 0 degrees to 45 degrees

Preferred starting position: See Figure 4-6.

End position: See Figure 4-7.

Goniometric alignment:

- Axis: Center over the anterior aspect of the hip joint at the anterior superior iliac spine (ASIS)

- Stationary arm: Align with an imaginary horizontal line, siting the ASIS of the opposite hip

- Moving arm: Align with the anterior midline of the femur, siting the center of the patella

Stabilization: The pelvis should be stabilized against a supporting surface. The clinician may use his/her hand on the lateral aspect of the knee to prevent hip rotation.

Substitutions: The subject may try to rotate the tested hip or bend laterally to the opposite side to increase the motion or avoid pain. He/she may also try to tilt the pelvis on the contralateral side.

Alternate method/position for testing: None.

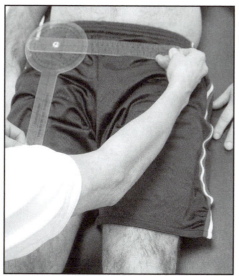

Figure 4-6. The subject should lie supine with the hip in midposition between flexion/extension and rotation.

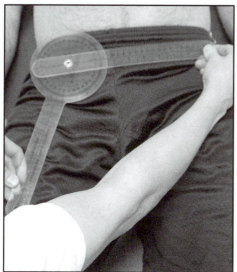

Figure 4-7. The hip should be in a position of maximal abduction at the end of the movement.

Hip Adduction

Planes/axis of movement: Movement occurs in the frontal plane around an anterior/posterior axis. This is the return motion from abduction.

Range of motion:

- 0 degrees to 30 degrees

Preferred starting position: See Figure 4-8.

End position: See Figure 4-9.

Goniometric alignment

- Axis: Center over the anterior aspect of the hip joint at the anterior superior iliac spine (ASIS)

- Stationary arm: Align with an imaginary horizontal line, siting the ASIS of the opposite hip

- Moving arm: Align with the anterior midline of the femur, siting the center of the patella

Stabilization: The pelvis should be stabilized against a supporting surface and encourage subject compliance to prevent ipsilateral tilting of the pelvis.

Substitutions: The subject may try to attempt to laterally flex the trunk toward the tested side to increase the range of motion or avoid pain with movement.

Alternate method/position for testing: None.

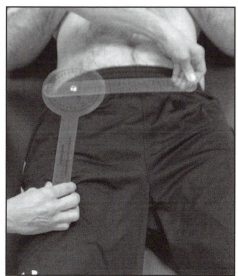

Figure 4-8. The subject lies in supine with the opposite lower extremity fully abducted to allow for full adduction of the tested limb. The hip should be in a neutral position between flexion/extension and rotation. The knee should be extended.

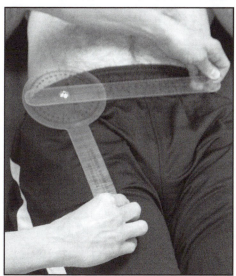

Figure 4-9. The tested hip should be in a position of maximal adduction at the end of the movement.

Hip Internal (Medial) Rotation

Planes/axis of movement: Movement occurs in the transverse plane around a longitudinal axis in the anatomic position and in the frontal plane around an anterior/posterior axis during testing.

Range of motion:

- 0 degrees to 45 degrees (with the hip flexed)
- 0 degrees to 30 degrees (with the hip extended)

Preferred starting position: See Figure 4-10.

End position: See Figure 4-11.

Goniometric alignment

- Axis: Center over the midpatellar surface
- Stationary arm: Align so the goniometer is perpendicular to the floor or parallel to the tabletop
- Moving arm: Align with the anterior midline of the lower leg, siting the midpoint between the two malleoli of the ankle

Stabilization: The distal end of the femur should be stabilized against a supporting surface through body weight. The clinician may have to use his/her hand to prevent hip adduction or flexion.

Substitutions: The subject may try to tilt the pelvis on the contralateral side or raise the pelvis off the table to gain increase the range of motion. He/she may also adduct the hip to avoid pain.

Alternate method/position for testing: See Figure 4-12.

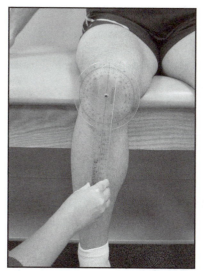

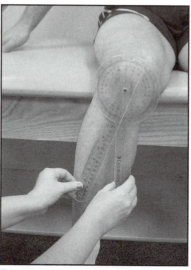

Figure 4-10. The subject should be in sitting on a tabletop with the hips and knees flexed to 90 degrees. The lower limb should hang freely over the edge of the table.

Figure 4-11. The hips should be in a position of maximal internal rotation at the end of the movement.

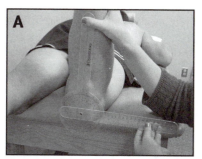

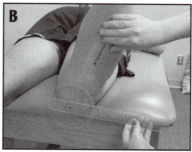

Figure 4-12. The subject may lie prone or supine with the hip in a neutral position with the knee flexed to 90 degrees. (A) Alternate starting position. (B) End position.

Hip External (Lateral) Rotation

Planes/axis of movement: Movement occurs in the transverse plane around a longitudinal axis in the anatomic position and in a frontal plane around an anterior/posterior axis during testing.

Range of motion:

- 0 degrees to 45 degrees (with the hip flexed)
- 0 degrees to 30 degrees (with the hip extended)

Preferred starting position: See Figure 4-13.

End position: See Figure 4-14.

Goniometric alignment:

- Axis: Center over the anterior midpatellar surface
- Stationary arm: Align so the goniometer is perpendicular to the floor or parallel to the tabletop
- Moving arm: Align with the anterior midline of the lower leg, siting the midpoint between the two malleoli of the ankle

Stabilization: The distal end of the femur should be stabilized against a supporting surface through body weight. The clinician may have to use his/her hand to prevent hip abduction or flexion.

Substitutions: See Figure 4-15.

Alternate method/position for testing: The subject may lie supine or prone with the hip in neutral with the knee flexed to 90 degrees.

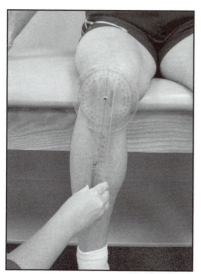

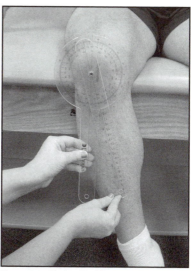

Figure 4-13. The subject should be sitting on a tabletop with the hips and knees flexed to 90 degrees. The lower limb should hang freely over the edge of the table.

Figure 4-14. The hip should be in a position of maximal external rotation at the end of the movement.

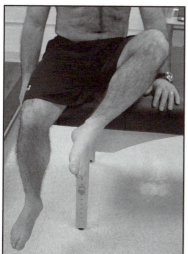

Figure 4-15. The subject may try to tilt or rotate the pelvis toward the ipsilateral side or raise the pelvis off the table to gain more range of motion. He/she may also try to abduct or flex the hip to avoid pain with movement.

THE KNEE (TIBIOFEMORAL JOINT)

Type of joint: The knee is a hinge joint with two degrees of freedom, allowing for flexion and extension with an axial rotation.

Capsular pattern: Flexion > extension.

Knee Flexion

Planes/axis of movement: Motion occurs in the sagittal plane around a coronal axis. Axial rotation occurs in the transverse plane when the knee is in a flexed position.

Range of motion:

- 0 degrees to 120 degrees (with the hip extended)
- 0 degrees to 135 degrees (with the hip flexed)

Preferred starting position: See Figure 4-16.

End position: See Figure 4-17.

Goniometric alignment:

- Axis: Center over the lateral epicondyle of the femur
- Stationary arm: Align with the lateral midline of the femur, siting the greater trochanter
- Moving arm: Align with the lateral midline of the fibula, siting the lateral malleolus

Stabilization: The pelvis should be stabilized against a supporting surface and the femur should be stabilized by the clinician's hand if necessary to prevent any hip movement.

Substitutions: The subject may try to rotate the hip to avoid pain.

Alternate method/position for testing: See Figure 4-18.

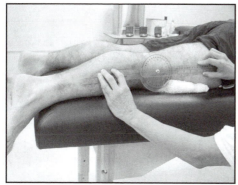

Figure 4-16. The subject is placed in prone with the hip in neutral position. The foot should be placed over the edge of the table-top. A folded towel should be placed under the anterior thigh to prevent compression on the patella.

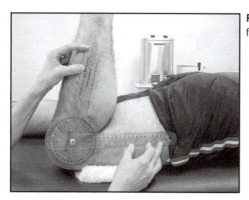

Figure 4-17. The knee should be maximally flexed at the end of the movement.

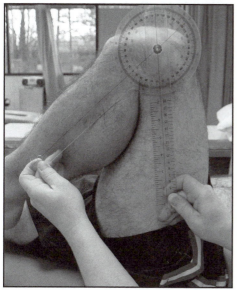

Figure 4-18. The subject may be placed supine with the hip flexed to 90 degrees or the subject may be placed in sidelying with the leg to be tested on the top. The knee and hip are both flexed in this position.

Knee Extension

Planes/axis of movement: Motion occurs in the sagittal plane around a coronal axis. Extension is the return motion from knee flexion.

Range of motion:

- 120 degrees to 0 degrees (from knee flexion with the hip extended)
- 135 degrees to 0 degrees (from knee flexion with the hip flexed)

Preferred starting position: See Figure 4-19.

End position: See Figure 4-20.

Goniometric alignment:

- Axis: Center over the lateral epicondyle of the femur
- Stationary arm: Align with the lateral midline of the femur, siting the greater trochanter
- Moving arm: Align with the lateral midline of the fibula, siting the lateral malleolus

Stabilization: The pelvis should be stabilized against a supporting surface and the femur should be stabilized by the clinician's hand if necessary to prevent any hip movement.

Substitutions: The subject may try to rotate the hip to avoid pain with movement.

Alternate method/position for testing: The subject may be placed in sidelying with the leg to be tested on top.

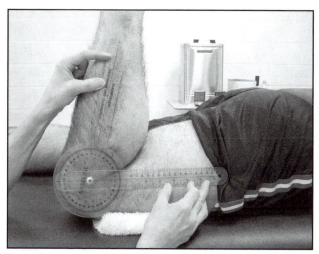

Figure 4-19. The subject is placed in prone with the hip in neutral position. A folded towel should be placed under the anterior thigh to prevent compression on the patella. The knee joint should be in a maximally flexed position.

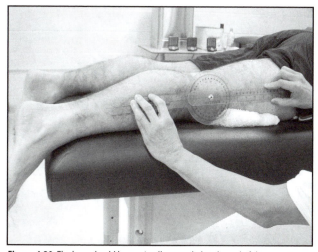

Figure 4-20. The knee should be maximally extended at the end of the movement.

TIBIAL TORSION

Tibial torsion is described as a slight lateral angulation of the distal tibia in comparison to the proximal aspect of the tibia. It may be assessed with a goniometer by measuring the angle of the malleoli to the talus.

Range of motion:

- 20 degrees to 30 degrees of torsion

Preferred starting position: See Figure 4-21 (in supine) and Figure 4-22 (in prone).

End position: See Figure 4-21 (in supine) and Figure 4-22 (in prone).

Goniometric alignment: A line should be drawn on the bottom of the heel horizontal to the tabletop. A second line is drawn on the bottom of the heel in line with both malleoli.

- Axis: Center over the intersection of the two lines
- Stationary arm: Align parallel to the tabletop in line with the horizontal line on the heel
- Moving arm: Align along the line connecting the two malleoli

Stabilization: The lower leg should be stabilized on a supporting surface.

Substitutions: The subject may move the lower limb during testing, which may cause an inaccurate measurement to be taken.

Alternate method/position for testing: The subject lies in prone with the knee flexed to 90 degrees.

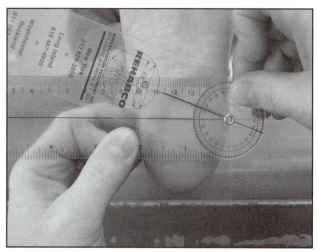

Figure 4-21. The subject may be positioned in supine or in prone. The foot should rest over the edge of the tabletop. The ankle and foot should be in a neutral position. The position remains the same throughout the measurement. Measurement shown in supine.

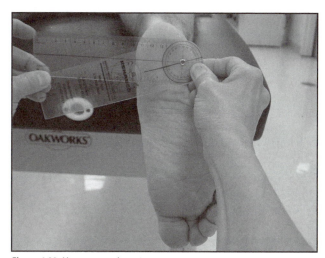

Figure 4-22. Measurement shown in prone.

THE ANKLE

Type of joint: Hinge joint with one degree of freedom. The axis of motion is obliquely oriented in the transverse plane and passes along a line that connects two points just distal to the tips of the malleoli. The movements of plantarflexion and dorsiflexion occur at this joint.

Capsular pattern: Plantarflexion > dorsiflexion.

Ankle Dorsiflexion

Planes/axis of movement: Motion occurs in the sagittal plane around a coronal axis.

Range of motion:

■ 0 degrees to 20 degrees

Preferred starting position: See Figure 4-23.

End position: See Figure 4-24.

Goniometric alignment:

■ Axis: Center over the lateral aspect of the lateral malleolus

■ Stationary arm: Align with the lateral midline of the fibula, siting the fibular head

■ Moving arm: Align with the lateral midline of the calcaneus

Stabilization: The tibia and fibula must be stabilized by the clinician (or on a supporting surface if the subject is in supine or prone) to prevent hip or knee motion.

Substitutions: The subject may try to flex the knee or hip to gain more range of motion or avoid pain during testing.

Alternate method/position for testing: See Figure 4-25.

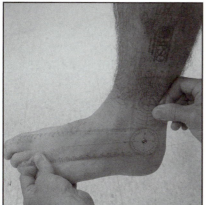

Figure 4-23. The subject is in sitting or supine with the knee flexed to at least 30 degrees. The foot should be in midposition between inversion and eversion. A towel roll is placed under the knee to maintain flexion.

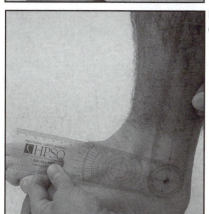

Figure 4-24. The ankle should be maximally dorsiflexed at the end of the movement.

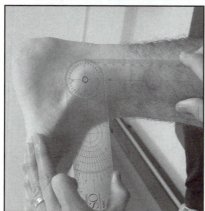

Figure 4-25. The subject may lie prone with the knee maintained in at least 30 degrees of flexion.

Ankle Plantarflexion

Planes/axis of movement: Motion occurs in the sagittal plane around a coronal axis.

Range of motion:

- 0 degrees to 45 degrees

Preferred starting position: See Figure 4-26.

End position: See Figure 4-27.

Goniometric alignment:

- Axis: Center over the lateral aspect of the lateral malleolus
- Stationary arm: Align with the lateral midline of the fibula, siting the fibular head
- Moving arm: Align parallel to the lateral midline of the calcaneus

Stabilization: The tibia and fibula must be stabilized by the clinician (or on a supporting surface if the subject is in supine or prone) to prevent knee or hip motion.

Substitutions: The subject may try to extend the knee or hip to gain more range of motion during testing.

Alternate method/position for testing: See Figure 4-28.

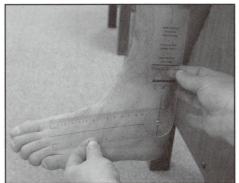

Figure 4-26. The subject is in sitting or supine with the knee flexed to at least 30 degrees. The foot should be in midposition between inversion and eversion. A towel roll is placed under the knee to maintain flexion.

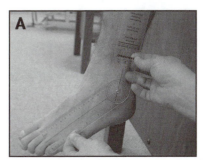
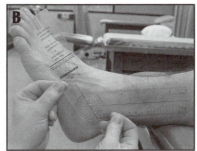

Figure 4-27. The ankle should be maximally plantarflexed at the end of the movement.

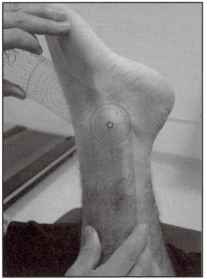

Figure 4-28. The subject may lie prone with the knee maintained in at least 30 degrees of flexion.

SUBTALAR JOINT (HINDFOOT)

Type of joint: The subtalar joint is a complex joint in which the inferior surface of the talus articulates with the calcaneus, navicular, and cuboid bones. Movement occurs along an oblique axis allowing for foot inversion and eversion. This axis is located along a line that originates on the lateral posterior aspect of the heel and continues in an anterior-superior medial direction.

Capsular pattern: None.

Subtalar Joint Inversion

Planes/axis of movement: This motion occurs in the frontal plane around an anterior/posterior axis in the anatomical position, but occurs in the transverse plane around a vertical axis during testing.

Range of motion:

- 0 degrees to 30 degrees

Preferred starting position: See Figure 4-29.

End position: See Figure 4-30.

Goniometric alignment:

- Axis: Center over the posterior aspect of the ankle midway between the malleoli
- Stationary arm: Align with the posterior midline of the lower leg
- Moving arm: Align with the posterior midline of the calcaneus

Stabilization: The lower leg must be stabilized on a supporting surface to prevent hip or knee motion.

Substitutions: The subject may try to rotate the hip or flex the knee to increase motion during testing.

Alternate method/position for testing: None.

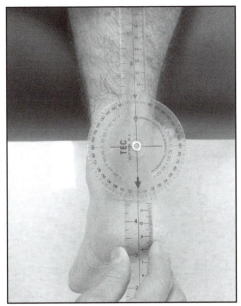

Figure 4-29. The subject is in prone with the hip in neutral position. The knee is in full extension with the foot over the edge of the supporting surface.

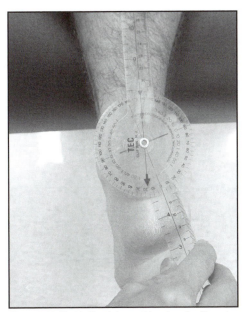

Figure 4-30. The hindfoot is in a position of maximal inversion at the end of the movement.

Subtalar Eversion

Planes/axis of movement: This motion occurs in the frontal plane around an anterior/posterior axis in the anatomical position, but occurs in the transverse plane around a vertical axis during testing.

Range of motion:

- 0 degrees to 25 degrees

Preferred starting position: See Figure 4-31.

End position: See Figure 4-32.

Goniometric alignment:

- Axis: Center over the posterior aspect of the ankle midway between the malleoli

- Stationary arm: Align with the posterior midline of the lower leg

- Moving arm: Align with the posterior midline of the calcaneus

Stabilization: The lower leg must be stabilized on a supporting surface to prevent knee and hip movement.

Substitutions: The subject may try to rotate the hip or flex the knee to increase the range of motion during testing.

Alternate method/position for testing: None.

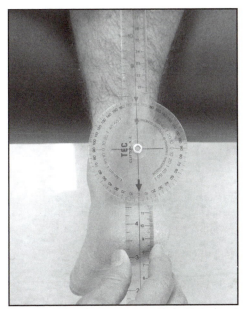

Figure 4-31. The subject is in prone with the hip in neutral position. The knee is in full extension with the foot over the edge of the supporting surface.

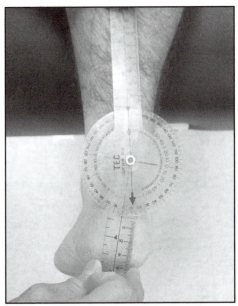

Figure 4-32. The hindfoot should be in a position of maximal eversion at the end of the movement.

TRANSVERSE TARSAL (MIDTARSAL) JOINT

Type of joint: This is a complex joint that involves the articulations of the talus and calcaneus proximally and the navicular and cuboid distally. The calcaneocuboid joint is saddle shaped and the talonavicular joint acts in a similar manner to a hinged type of joint, with the convex surface of the talus articulating with the concave surface of the navicular. The movements of midfoot inversion and eversion occur at this joint.

There is also motion that exists between the midfoot and forefoot which includes movements that occur at the tarsometatarsal joints. These are the articulations between the cuboid and three cuneiform bones with the bases of the five metatarsals. A slight amount of flexion and extension occurs with some rotary motion around the metatarsal joints, allowing the foot to move in an arc fashion.

Capsular pattern: None.

Midtarsal Inversion

Planes/axis of movement: Movement is a combination of supination, adduction, and plantarflexion. The motion is measured in the frontal plane around an anterior/posterior axis because of the limitation of the goniometer to measure in a singular plane.

Range of motion:

- 0 degrees to 30 degrees

Preferred starting position: See Figure 4-33.

End position: See Figure 4-34.

Goniometric alignment:

- Axis: Center over the anterior aspect of the ankle midway between the malleoli
- Stationary arm: Align along the anterior midline of the tibial crest, siting the tibial tuberosity
- Moving arm: Align along the dorsal aspect of the second metatarsal shaft

Stabilization: The lower leg should be stabilized by the clinician (or on a supporting surface if the subject is in supine).

Substitutions: The subject may try to rotate the hip and knee to increase the range of motion during testing.

Alternate method/position for testing: See Figure 4-35.

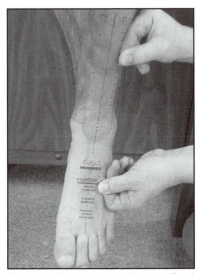

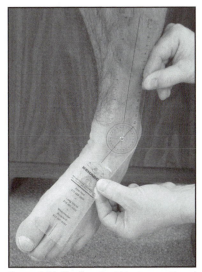

Figure 4-33. The subject sits with the knee flexed to 90 degrees.

Figure 4-34. The foot should be in a position of maximal inversion at the end of the movement.

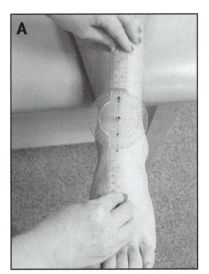

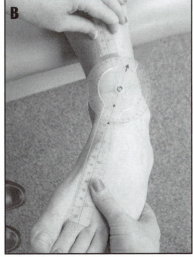

Figure 4-35. The subject may also be placed in supine with the hip and knee in extension and in neutral rotation. (A) Alternate starting position. (B) End position.

Midtarsal Eversion

Planes/axis of movement: Movement is a combination of pronation, abduction, and dorsiflexion. Motion is measured in the frontal plane around an anterior/posterior axis because of the limitation of the goniometer to measure in a singular plane.

Range of motion:

- 0 degrees to 25 degrees

Preferred starting position: See Figure 4-36.

End position: See Figure 4-37.

Goniometric alignment:

- Axis: Center over the anterior aspect of the ankle midway between the malleoli

- Stationary arm: Align along the anterior midline of the tibial crest, siting the tibial tuberosity

- Moving arm: Align along the dorsal aspect of the second metatarsal shaft

Stabilization: The lower leg should be stabilized by the clinician (or on a supporting surface if the subject is in supine).

Substitutions: The subject may try to rotate the hip or knee to increase the range of motion during testing.

Alternate method/position for testing: See Figure 4-38.

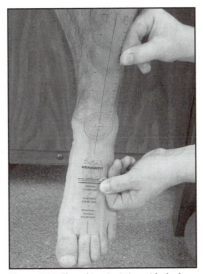

Figure 4-36. The subject is sitting with the knee flexed to 90 degrees.

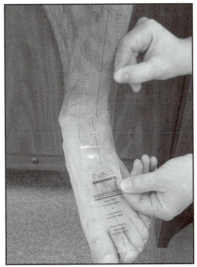

Figure 4-37. The foot should be in a position of maximal eversion at the end of the movement.

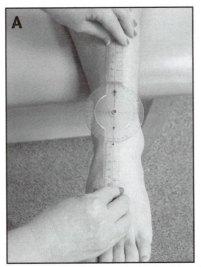

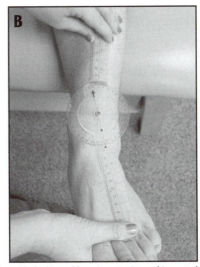

Figure 4-38. The subject may also be placed in supine with the hip and knee in extension and in neutral position. (A) Alternate starting position. (B) End position.

THE FIRST TOE
(METATARSOPHALANGEAL JOINTS)

Type of joint: These joints are of the condyloid type and allow for two degrees of freedom, allowing for flexion/extension and abduction/adduction movements.

Capsular pattern: Great toe – extension > flexion.

MTP Flexion

Planes/axis of movement: Motion occurs in the sagittal plane around a coronal axis.

Range of motion:

- 0 degrees to 45 degrees

Preferred starting position: See Figure 4-39.

End position: See Figure 4-40.

Goniometric alignment:

- Axis: Center over the dorsal aspect of the first MTP joint

- Stationary arm: Align along the dorsal midline of the shaft of the first metatarsal

- Moving arm: Align along the dorsal midline of the proximal phalanx

Stabilization: The lower leg should be stabilized on a supporting surface and first metatarsal of the foot should be stabilized.

Substitutions: The subject may try to attempt to plantarflex the ankle to increase the range of motion during testing.

Alternate method/position for testing: None.

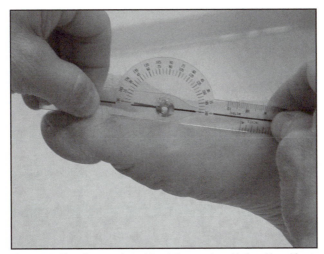

Figure 4-39. The subject may be in either sitting or supine with the ankle and foot in a neutral position over the edge of a table.

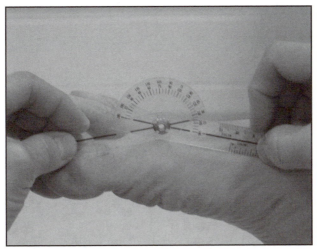

Figure 4-40. The first MTP joint should be in maximal flexion at the end of the movement.

MTP Extension/Hyperextension

Planes/axis of movement: Motion occurs in the sagittal plane around a coronal axis. Extension of the MTP joint is the return motion from MTP flexion.

Range of motion:

- 45 degrees to 0 degrees of extension

- 0 degrees to 90 degrees of hyperextension

Preferred starting position: See Figure 4-41.

End position: See Figure 4-42.

Goniometric alignment:

- Axis: Center over the dorsal aspect of the first MTP joint

- Stationary arm: Align along the dorsal midline of the shaft of the first metatarsal

- Moving arm: Align along the dorsal midline of the proximal phalanx

Stabilization: The lower leg should be stabilized on a supporting surface and the first metatarsal of the foot should be stabilized.

Substitutions: The subject may attempt to dorsiflex the ankle to increase the range of motion during testing.

Alternate method/position for testing: See Figure 4-43.

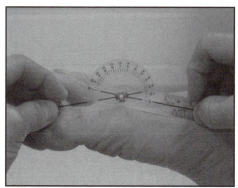

Figure 4-41. The subject may be in sitting or supine with the ankle and foot in neutral position over the edge of a table. The first MTP joint should be in full flexion.

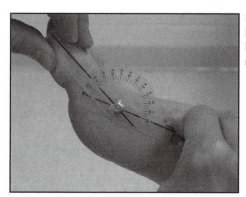

Figure 4-42. The first MTP joint should be in a position of maximal extension/hyperextension at the end of the movement.

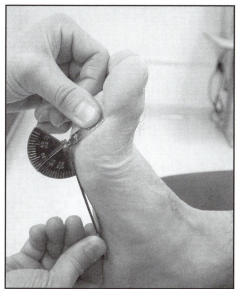

Figure 4-43. This motion may also be measured on the plantar surface of the first MTP joint.

MTP Abduction

Planes/axis of movement: Motion occurs in the transverse plane around a vertical axis in the anatomical position.

Range of motion:

■ The range of motion of the tested toe should be equal when compared to the nontested toe

Preferred starting position: See Figure 4-44.

End position: See Figure 4-45.

Goniometric alignment:

■ Axis: Center over the dorsal aspect of the first MTP joint

■ Stationary arm: Align with the dorsal midline of the first metatarsal

■ Moving arm: Align with the dorsal midline of the proximal phalanx

Stabilization: The first metatarsal should be stabilized to prevent inversion or eversion of the foot.

Substitutions: The subject may try to invert the foot to avoid pain with motion.

Alternate method/position for testing: None.

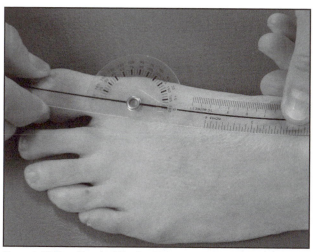

Figure 4-44. The subject should be placed in sitting or supine with the ankle and foot in neutral position between inversion and eversion. The MTP and IP joints should be in a neutral position between flexion and extension.

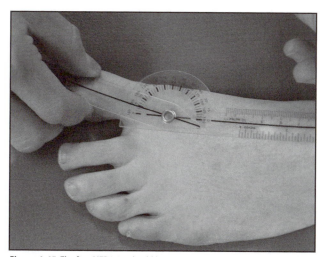

Figure 4-45. The first MTP joint should be in a position of maximal abduction at the end of the movement.

THE FIRST TOE (INTERPHALANGEAL JOINT)

Type of joint: Hinge joint with one degree of freedom, allowing for flexion and extension only.

Capsular pattern: Flexion > extension.

IP Flexion

Planes/axis of movement: Motion occurs in the sagittal plane around a coronal axis.

Range of motion:

- 0 degrees to 90 degrees

Preferred starting position: See Figure 4-46.

End position: See Figure 4-47.

Goniometric alignment:

- Axis: Align over the dorsal aspect of the IP joint
- Stationary arm: Align along the dorsal midline of the shaft of the proximal phalanx
- Moving arm: Align over the dorsal midline of the shaft of the distal phalanx

Stabilization: The lower leg should be stabilized on a supporting surface and the proximal phalanx should be stabilized.

Substitutions: The subject may try to plantarflex the ankle during testing to increase the range of motion.

Alternate method/position for testing: None.

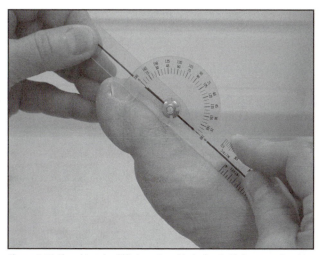

Figure 4-46. The subject should lie in supine with the foot/ankle in a neutral position over the edge of a table.

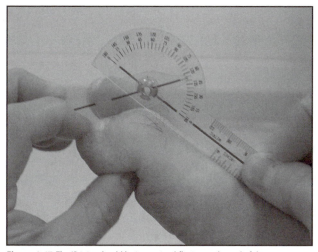

Figure 4-47. The IP joint should be in maximal flexion at the end of the movement.

IP Extension/Hyperextension

Planes/axis of movement: Motion occurs in the sagittal plane around a coronal axis.

Range of motion:

- 90 degrees to 0 degrees; hyperextension is minimal

Preferred starting position: See Figure 4-48.

End position: See Figure 4-49.

Goniometric alignment:

- Axis: Align over the dorsal aspect of the IP joint
- Stationary arm: Align over the dorsal midline of the shaft of the proximal phalanx
- Moving arm: Align over the dorsal midline of the shaft of the distal phalanx

Stabilization: The lower leg should be stabilized on a supporting surface and the proximal phalanx should be stabilized.

Substitutions: The subject may try to dorsiflex the ankle during testing to gain more range of motion.

Alternate method/position for testing: See Figure 4-50.

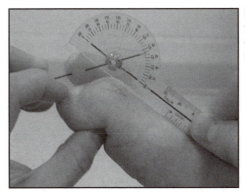

Figure 4-48. The subject should lie supine with the foot/ankle in a neutral position over the edge of a table. The IP joint should be in full flexion.

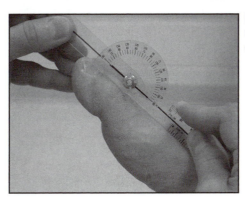

Figure 4-49. The IP joint should be in maximal extension/hyperextension at the end of the movement.

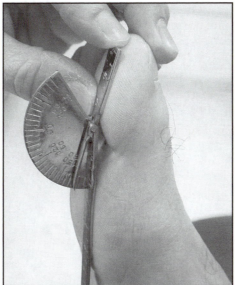

Figure 4-50. The goniometer may be placed on the plantar surface of the IP joint to measure hyperextension.

THE FOUR LATERAL TOES (METATARSOPHALANGEAL JOINTS)

Type of joint: Hinge joint with one degree of freedom, allowing for flexion and extension only.

Capsular pattern: Flexion > extension.

MTP Flexion

Planes/axis of movement: Motion occurs in the sagittal plane around a coronal axis.

Range of motion:

- 0 degrees to 40 degrees

Preferred starting position: See Figure 4-51.

End position: See Figure 4-52.

Goniometric alignment:

- Axis: Center over the dorsal aspect of the tested MTP joint
- Stationary arm: Align over the dorsal midline of the metatarsal bone
- Moving arm: Align over the dorsal midline of the proximal phalanx

Stabilization: The metatarsals must be stabilized to prevent foot and ankle movement.

Substitutions: The subject may attempt to plantarflex the ankle to avoid pain with testing or increase the range of motion.

Alternate method/position for testing: None.

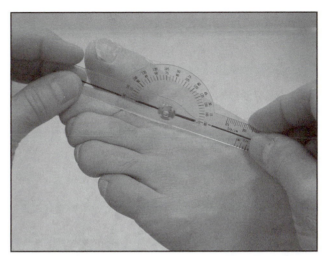

Figure 4-51. The subject should lie in supine with the foot/ankle in a neutral position over the edge of a table.

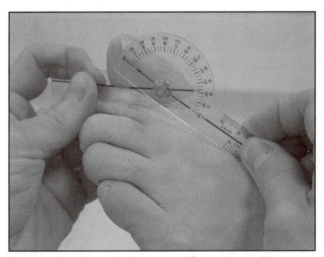

Figure 4-52. The MTP joint should be in maximal flexion at the end of the motion.

MTP Extension/Hyperextension

Planes/axis of movement: This is the return motion from MTP flexion. Motion occurs in the sagittal plane around a coronal axis. The proximal phalanx glides dorsally on the metatarsal.

Range of motion:

- 40 degrees to 0 degrees (extension)
- 0 degrees to 45 (hyperextension)

Preferred starting position: See Figure 4-53.

End position: See Figure 4-54.

Goniometric alignment:

- Axis: Center over the dorsal aspect of the testing MTP joint
- Stationary arm: Align over the dorsal midline of the metatarsal bone
- Moving arm: Align over the dorsal midline of the proximal phalanx

Stabilization: The metatarsals must be stabilized to prevent foot and ankle movement.

Substitutions: The subject may attempt to dorsiflex the ankle to avoid pain with testing or increase the range of motion.

Alternate method/position for testing: See Figure 4-55.

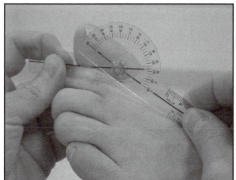

Figure 4-53. The subject lies supine with the foot/ankle in a neutral position over the edge of a table. The MTP joint should be in full flexion.

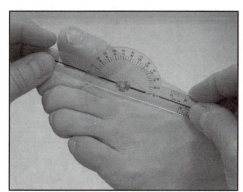

Figure 4-54. The MTP joint should be in a position of maximal extension at the end of the movement.

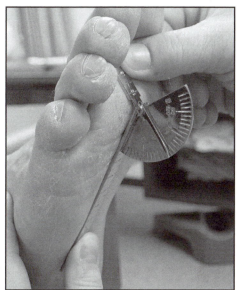

Figure 4-55. The goniometer may be placed on the plantar surface of the MTP joint to measure hyperextension.

THE FOUR LATERAL TOES (PROXIMAL INTERPHALANGEAL JOINTS)

Type of joint: These joints are hinge joints with one degree of freedom, allowing for flexion and extension only.

Capsular pattern: Flexion > extension.

PIP Flexion

Planes/axis of movement: Motion occurs in the sagittal plane around a coronal axis.

Range of motion:

■ 0 degrees to 35 degrees for the four lateral toes

Preferred starting position: See Figure 4-56.

End position: See Figure 4-57.

Goniometric alignment:

■ Axis: Center over the dorsal aspect of the PIP joint

■ Stationary arm: Align along the dorsal midline of the shaft of the proximal phalanx

■ Moving arm: Align along the dorsal midline of the shaft of the middle phalanx

Stabilization: The proximal phalanx and metatarsals of the foot should be stabilized.

Substitutions: The subject may try to plantarflex the ankle during testing to increase the range of motion.

Alternate method/position for testing: None.

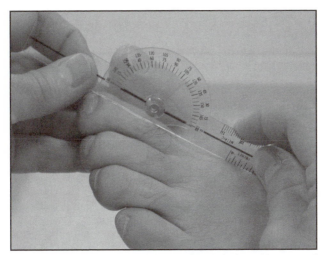

Figure 4-56. The subject may be sitting or supine with the foot/ankle in a neutral position over the edge of a table.

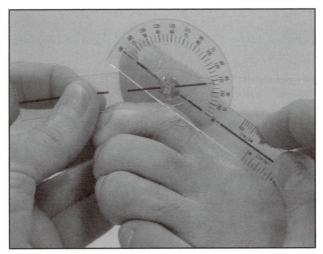

Figure 4-57. The PIP joint being tested should be in a position of maximal flexion at the end of the movement.

PIP Extension

Planes/axis of movement: Motion occurs in the sagittal plane around a coronal axis.

Range of motion:

- 35 degrees to 0 degrees; hyperextension is minimal

Preferred starting position: See Figure 4-58.

End position: See Figure 4-59.

Goniometric alignment:

- Axis: Center over the dorsal aspect of the PIP joint

- Stationary arm: Align along the dorsal midline of the shaft of the proximal phalanx

- Moving arm: Align along the dorsal midline of the shaft of the middle phalanx

Stabilization: The proximal phalanx and metatarsals of the foot should be stabilized.

Substitutions: The subject may try to dorsiflex the ankle during testing in an attempt to increase the range of motion.

Alternate method/position for testing: None.

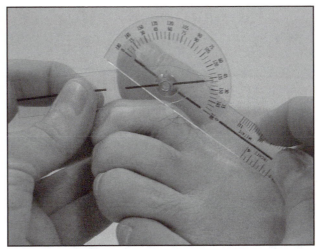

Figure 4-58. The subject may be in sitting or supine with the foot/ankle in a neutral position over the edge of a table. The PIP joint should be in full flexion.

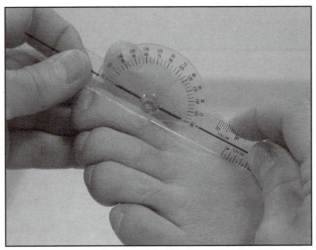

Figure 4-59. The PIP joint being tested should be in a position of maximal extension at the end of the movement.

THE FOUR LATERAL TOES (DISTAL INTERPHALANGEAL JOINTS)

Type of joint: These joints are hinge joints with one degree of freedom, allowing for flexion and extension only.

Capsular pattern: Flexion > extension.

DIP Flexion

Planes/axis of movement: The motion occurs in the sagittal plane around a coronal axis.

Range of motion:

- 0 degrees to 60 degrees

Preferred starting position: See Figure 4-60.

End position: See Figure 4-61.

Goniometric alignment:

- Axis: Center over the dorsal aspect of the DIP joint
- Stationary arm: Align along the dorsal midline of the shaft of the middle phalanx
- Moving arm: Align along the dorsal midline of the shaft of the distal phalanx

Stabilization: The middle and proximal phalanges should be stabilized.

Substitutions: The subject may attempt to plantarflex the ankle or flex the MTP or PIP joints to increase the range of motion.

Alternate method/position for testing: None.

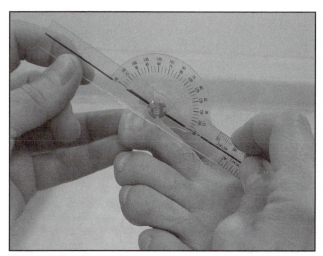

Figure 4-60. The subject may be in sitting or supine with the foot/ankle in a neutral position over the edge of a table.

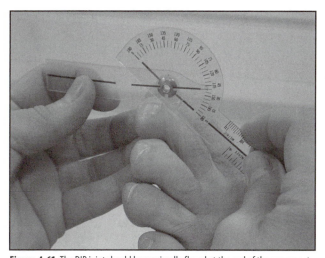

Figure 4-61. The DIP joint should be maximally flexed at the end of the movement.

DIP Extension

Planes/axis of movement: Movement occurs in the sagittal plane around a coronal axis.

Range of motion:

- 60 degrees to 0 degrees; hyperextension is minimal

Preferred starting position: See Figure 4-62.

End position: See Figure 4-63.

Goniometric alignment:

- Axis: Center over the dorsal aspect of the DIP joint
- Stationary arm: Align over the dorsal midline of the middle phalanx
- Moving arm: Align over the dorsal midline of the distal phalanx

Stabilization: The middle and proximal phalanges should be stabilized.

Substitutions: The subject may attempt to dorsiflex the ankle or extend the MTP or PIP joints during testing to increase the range of motion.

Alternate method/position for testing: None.

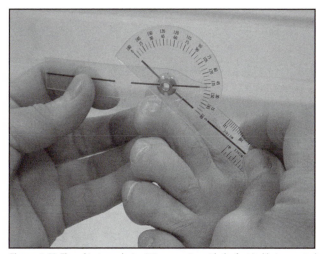

Figure 4-62. The subject may be in sitting or supine with the foot/ankle in a neutral position over the edge of a table. The DIP joint should be in full flexion.

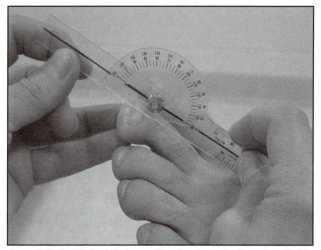

Figure 4-63. The DIP should be in a position of maximal extension at the end of the movement.

SECTION V

TMJ Joint

L. Van Ost
Cram Session in Goniometry:
A Handbook for Students & Clinicians (pp. 151-157)
© 2010 SLACK Incorporated

THE TEMPOROMANDIBULAR JOINT

Type of joint: This is a complex joint that allows for opening, closing, protrusion, retrusion, and lateral deviation of the jaw. The TMJ is composed of the mandibular condyle and articulating surface of the glenoid fossa of the temporal bone. Between the mandibular condyle and glenoid fossa is an articulating disc or meniscus. During the opening of jaw, a hinge type of motion is followed by a gliding motion of the condyle and the condyle moves down and out of the glenoid fossa on the disc. The disc then moves forward on the tubercle of the zygomatic process to complete the motion.

Capsular pattern: Restrictions in the ability to open the mouth.

Depression of the Mandible (Opening of the Mouth)

Planes/axis of movement: Motion occurs in the sagittal plane around a coronal axis.

Range of motion:

- Approximately 2 inches or 3.5 to 4.0 cm; also equal to the width of three fingers between the teeth

Preferred starting position: The subject should be in sitting with the cervical spine in neutral.

End position: See Figure 5-1.

Measurement of motion: The movement is measured with a tape measure or ruler. The distance between the upper central incisor teeth and lower central incisor teeth is recorded.

Stabilization: The head and neck should be stabilized to prevent motion of the cervical spine during testing.

Substitutions: The subject may try to flex the cervical spine or retract the head to increase the range of motion or avoid pain during testing.

Alternate method/position for testing: None.

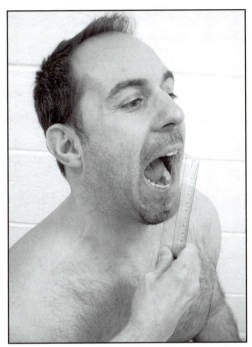

Figure 5-1. The subject should be in sitting with the cervical spine in neutral. The mouth should be open as far as possible at end of the motion.

Anterior Protrusion of the Mandible

Planes/axis of movement: Motion occurs in the transverse plane and is a translatory type of motion.

Range of motion:

- Normal motion is the ability of the lower central incisor teeth to move forward beyond the upper central incisor teeth

Preferred starting position: The subject should be in sitting with the cervical spine in a neutral position.

End position: See Figure 5-2.

Measurement of motion: The movement is measured with a tape measure or ruler. The distance between the lower central incisor teeth and upper central incisor teeth is measured.

Stabilization: The head and neck should be stabilized to prevent motion of the cervical spine during testing.

Substitutions: The subject may attempt to extend the cervical spine or protrude the head to avoid pain or increase the range of motion during testing.

Alternate method/position for testing: None.

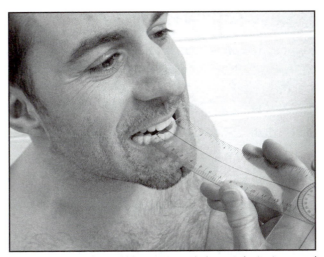

Figure 5-2. The subject should be in sitting with the cervical spine in a neutral position. The mandible should be protruded as far as possible at the end of the movement.

Lateral Protrusion of the Mandible

Planes/axis of movement: Motion occurs in the transverse plane and is a translatory type of motion.

Range of motion:

- Normal amount of motion allows for a comparable amount of lateral motion to both the right and left sides

Preferred starting position: The subject should be sitting with cervical spine in a neutral position.

End position: See Figure 5-3.

Measurement of motion: The movement is measured with a tape measure or ruler. The distance between the most lateral points of the lower and upper cuspid teeth or first bicuspid teeth are recorded.

Stabilization: The head and neck should be stabilized to prevent motion of the cervical spine during testing.

Substitutions: The subject may try to rotate the cervical spine to avoid pain or increase the range of motion during testing.

Alternate method/position for testing: None.

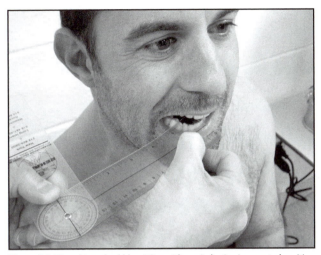

Figure 5-3. The subject should be sitting with cervical spine in a neutral position. The mandible should be in a position of maximal lateral protrusion at the end of the movement.

Appendices

APPENDIX A: GENERAL PROCEDURE FOR GONIOMETRIC MEASUREMENT

- The subject should be placed in a position closely correlating to the anatomical position in order to place the joints in a zero starting position and to provide proper stabilization. It is important to attempt to position the subject in the same way each time the measurement is taken to ensure reliable results. The subject should be properly dressed in order to fully visualize the limb and allow free movement.

- It is important to explain the procedure to the subject and demonstrate the movement to ensure proper motion during measurement. Take a visual estimate to get an idea of the joint's range of motion.

- Make sure the proximal limb segment is stabilized to prevent substitution and inaccurate readings.

- Locate and, if necessary, mark the appropriate anatomic landmarks to help ensure proper alignment of the goniometer.

- Find the approximate axis of the joint being measured and place the fulcrum of the goniometer at this point.

- Align the stationary arm parallel to the longitudinal axis of the proximal portion of the limb segment and the movable arm parallel to the longitudinal axis of the distal limb segment, siting the appropriate landmarks. Keep in mind that it might be necessary to reverse the stationary arm to align it with the distal limb segment and align the movable arm with the proximal limb segment if the subject position or the goniometer itself does not allow for a proper reading. Proper alignment of the arms of the goniometer will ensure proper alignment of the fulcrum.

- Do not press the goniometer against the limb as this might distort the reading. Hold the arms with the thumb and first two fingers in order to clearly see the readings.

- Take the first reading at the beginning of the motion. Remove the goniometer. Allow the motion to occur (either actively or passively) and realign the goniometer at the end of the motion. Do not move the stationary arm that is aligned against the proximal body segment.

- If the subject has no limitations and is in the recommended testing position, assume the starting point is zero degrees. The end point of the motion is recorded in a positive number away from zero. If there is an impairment and the movement does not start at zero, record the amount of limitation in degrees.

APPENDIX B: COMMONLY USED TERMS IN GONIOMETRY

abduction: Motion at a joint so that the distal segment is moved laterally away from the midline of the body.

adduction: Motion at a joint so that the distal segment is moved medially toward the midline of the body.

axis of rotation: A line at right angles to the plane in which adjacent limb segments move and about which all moving parts of the segments rotate in a circular path. Otherwise known as the "fulcrum," this is the point where both arms of the goniometer meet the on the body of the protractor. It is identifiable by the rivet or tension knob connecting the two arms together. The axis of the goniometer should coincide with the axis of the joint being tested.

deviation: Moving away from a starting position; frequently to denote abduction or adduction relative to the midline or rotation from a starting point.

dorsiflexion: Flexing or bending of the foot toward the leg so that the angle between the dorsum of the foot and the leg is decreased.

eversion: Turning outward; turning the sole of the foot so it faces laterally.

extension: Movement of a joint so that the two adjacent segments are moved apart and the joint angle is increased.

flexion: Movement of a joint so the two adjacent segments approach each other and the joint angle is decreased.

fluid goniometer: Consists of a 360-degree scale in a flat, fluid-filled circular tube that contains a small air bubble. The device is attached to or placed onto the limb or body part, and as the limb/body part moves, the scale rotates and the bubble remains stationary. The range of motion is read at the point the scale stops moving.

frontal or coronal planes: A vertical plane at right angles to the sagittal plane, dividing the body into ventral and dorsal halves.

goniometer: An instrument used to measure the joint movement and joint angles of the body.

goniometry: Derived from the Greek words "gonia," meaning angle, and "metron," meaning measure. The measurement of angles of the human body.

horizontal or transverse plane: Any plane through the body that divides the body into upper and lower halves.

inversion: Turning inward; turning the sole of the foot so it faces medially.

lateral (external) rotation: The rotation of a joint segment in the transverse plane around a vertical or longitudinal axis away from the midline of the body or toward the posterior surface of the body.

longitudinal axis: A line passing through a bone or segment, around which the parts are symmetrically arranged and lying in both the frontal and sagittal planes.

medial (internal) rotation: The rotation of a joint segment in the transverse plane around a vertical or longitudinal axis toward the midline of the body or toward the anterior surface of the body.

moving arm: The arm of the goniometer that is movable and is aligned with the segment that is distal to the joint being measured.

opposition: Moving the thumb away from the palm in a direction perpendicular to the plane of the hand allowing the thumb to touch the pad of the fifth digit.

plantarflexion: Flexing or bending of the foot in the direction of the sole so that the angle between the dorsum of the foot and leg is increased.

pronation: Rotating of the forearm so the palm of the hand is down or posterior in the anatomical position.

rotation: The turning or moving of a part around a fixed axis in a curved path.

sagittal plane: The vertical, anterior-posterior plane through the longitudinal axis of the trunk, dividing the body into right and left halves.

stationary arm: The arm of the goniometer that is fixed and aligned in parallel with the longitudinal axis of the segment proximal to the joint being measured.

substitution: A movement performed by the subject in an attempt to avoid pain caused by testing or to increase the joint range of motion.

supination: Rotating the forearm so the palm of the hand is up or anterior in the anatomical position.

universal goniometer: A plastic or metal device that consists of a protractor connected to two arms, one of which is attached to the body by a rivet. This is the most common type of goniometer used in the clinical setting.

APPENDIX C: NORMAL RANGE OF MOTION VALUES IN ADULTS

JOINT	AAOS	BOONE & AZEN	DANIELS & WORTHINGHAM	HOPPENFELD
SHOULDER				
Flexion	180	167	90	90
Extension	60	62	50	45
Abduction	180	184	90	180
Internal rotation	70	69	90	55
External rotation	90	104	90	45
Horizontal abduction	45	45	-----	-----
Horizontal adduction	135	140	-----	-----
ELBOW				
Flexion	150	143	160	150
RADIOULNAR				
Pronation	80	76	90	90
Supination	80	82	90	90
WRIST				
Flexion	80	76	90	80
Extension	70	75	70	70
Radial deviation	20	22	25	20
Ulnar deviation	30	36	65	30
THUMB—CMC				
Abduction	70	-----	50	70
Flexion	15	-----	-----	-----
Extension	20	-----	-----	-----
Opposition	Thumb tip to tip of 5th digit	-----	Thumb tip to tip of 5th digit	Thumb tip to tip of 5th digit
THUMB—MCP				
Flexion	50	-----	70	50
THUMB—IP				
Flexion	80	-----	90	90
DIGITS II-V—MCP				
Flexion	90	-----	90	90
Extension	45	-----	30	45
Abduction	-----	-----	25	20
DIGITS II-V—PIP				
Flexion	100	-----	120	100
DIGITS II-V—DIP				
Flexion	90	-----	80	90
Extension	-----	-----	-----	10

JOINT	KAPANJI	GERHARDT & RUSSE	AOA	DORINSON & WAGNER	KENDALL, KENDALL, & WADSWORTH
SHOULDER					
Flexion	180	170	-----	180	180
Extension	50	50	-----	45	45
Abduction	180	170	-----	180	180
Internal rotation	95	80	-----	90	70
External rotation	80	90	-----	90	90
Horizontal abduction	-----	30	-----	-----	-----
Horizontal adduction	-----	135	-----	-----	-----
ELBOW					
Flexion	145	150	146	150	145
RADIOULNAR					
Pronation	85	80	71	80	90
Supination	90	90	84	70	90
WRIST					
Flexion	85	60	73	80	80
Extension	85	50	71	55	70
Radial deviation	15	20	19	20	20
Ulnar deviation	-----	30	33	40	35
THUMB—CMC					
Abduction	-----	-----	-----	80	-----
Flexion	-----	-----	-----	50	-----
Extension	-----	-----	-----	50	-----
Opposition	-----	-----	-----	Thumb tip to tip of 5th digit	-----
THUMB—MCP					
Flexion	-----	-----	-----	80	-----
THUMB—IP					
Flexion	-----	-----	-----	90	-----
DIGITS II-V—MCP					
Flexion	-----	-----	-----	-----	-----
Extension	-----	-----	-----	-----	-----
Abduction	-----	-----	-----	-----	-----
DIGITS II-V—PIP					
Flexion	-----	-----	-----	100	-----
DIGITS II-V—DIP					
Flexion	-----	-----	-----	80	-----
Extension	-----	-----	-----	-----	-----

JOINT	AAOS	BOONE & AZEN	DANIELS & WORTHINGHAM	HOPPENFELD
HIP				
Flexion	120	122	125	135
Extension	30	10	15	30
Abduction	45	46	45	50
Adduction	30	27	0	30
Internal rotation	45	47	45	35
External rotation	45	47	45	45
KNEE				
Flexion	135	143	130	135
ANKLE				
Dorsiflexion	20	13	-----	20
Plantarflexion	50	56	45	50
SUBTALAR JOINT				
Inversion	35	37	-----	5
Eversion	15	26	-----	5
TRANSVERSE TARSAL				
Inversion	20	-----	-----	20
Eversion	10	-----	-----	10
FIRST TOE—MTP				
Flexion	45	-----	-----	45
Extension	70	-----	-----	90
FIRST TOE—IP				
Flexion	90	-----	-----	-----
TOES II-V—MTP				
Flexion	40	-----	35	-----
Extension	40	-----	-----	-----
TOES II-V—PIP				
Flexion	35	-----	90	-----
TOES II-V—DIP				
Flexion	-----	-----	-----	-----

Joint	Kapanji	Gerhardt & Russe	AOA	Dorinson & Wagner	Kendall, Kendall, & Wadsworth
Hip					
Flexion	120	125	-----	-----	125
Extension	30	15	-----	-----	10
Abduction	30	45	-----	-----	45
Adduction	30	15	-----	-----	-----
Internal rotation	30	45	-----	-----	-----
External rotation	60	45	-----	-----	-----
Knee					
Flexion	160	130	134	-----	140
Ankle					
Dorsiflexion	30	20	18	-----	20
Plantarflexion	50	45	48	-----	45
Subtalar Joint					
Inversion	52	40	5	-----	-----
Eversion	30	20	5	-----	-----
Transverse Tarsal					
Inversion	-----	-----	-----	50	-----
Eversion	-----	-----	-----	20	-----
First Toe—MTP					
Flexion	-----	-----	-----	-----	30
Extension	-----	-----	-----	-----	40
First Toe—IP					
Flexion	-----	-----	-----	-----	-----
Toes II-V—MTP					
Flexion	-----	-----	-----	-----	-----
Extension	-----	-----	-----	-----	-----
Toes II-V—PIP					
Flexion	-----	-----	-----	-----	-----
Toes II-V—DIP					
Flexion	-----	-----	-----	-----	-----

APPENDIX D: ANATOMICAL ZERO

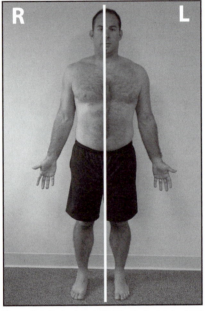

Figure D-1. Sagittal plane (divides the body into right/left).

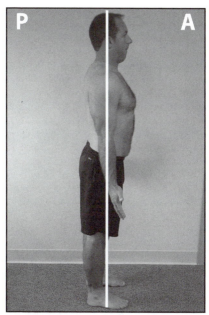

Figure D-2. Frontal plane (divides the body into anterior/posterior).

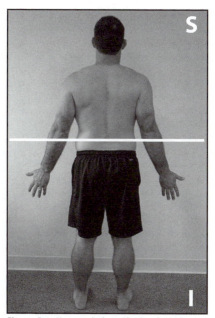

Figure D-3. Horizontal plane (divides the body into superior/inferior).

BIBLIOGRAPHY

American Academy of Orthopaedic Surgeons. *Joint Motion: Method of Measuring and Recording.* Chicago, IL: American Academy of Orthopaedic Surgeons; 1965.

American Orthopaedic Association. *The Manual of Orthopaedic Surgery.* Chicago, IL: American Orthopaedic Association; 1972.

Boone DC, Azen SP. Normal range of motion of joints in male subjects. *J Bone Joint Surg Am.* 1979;61:756-759.

Clark WA. A system of joint measurement. *J Orthop Surg.* 1920;2:687-700.

Clarkson HM. *Joint Motion and Functional Assessment: A Research-Based Practical Guide.* Philadelphia, PA: Lippincott Williams & Wilkins; 2005.

Daniels L, Worthingham C. *Manual Muscle Testing: Techniques of Manual Examination.* 3rd ed. Philadelphia, PA: WB Saunders; 1972.

Dorinson SM, Wagner ML. An exact technique for clinically measuring and recording joint motion. *Arch Phys Med.* 1948;29:468-475.

Elveru RA, Rothstein JM, Lamb RL, Riddle DL. Methods for taking subtalar joint measurements: a clinical report. *Phys Ther.* 1988;68: 678-682.

Eyadah AA, Ivanova MK. Methods for measurement of tibial torsion. *Kuwait Medical Journal.* 2001;33 (1): 3-6.

Fitzgerald GK, Wynveen KJ, Rheault W, Rothschild B. Objective assessment with establishment of normal values for lumbar spinal range of motion. *Phys Ther.* 1983;63(11): 1776-1781.

Gerhardt JJ, Cocchiarella L, Lea RD. *The Practical Guide to Range of Motion Assessment.* Chicago, IL: American Medical Association Press; 2002.

Gerhardt JJ, Russe OA. *International SFTR Method of Measuring and Recording Joint Motion.* Bern, Germany: Hans Huber; 1975.

Greene WB, Heckman JD, eds. *The Clinical Measurement of Joint Motion.* Rosemont, IL: American Academy of Orthopaedic Surgeons; 1994.

Griffin LY. *Essentials of Musculoskeletal Care.* 3rd ed. Rosemont, IL: American Academy of Orthopaedic Surgeons; 2005.

Hellebrandt FA, Duvall E, Moore ML. The measurement of joint motion. Reliability of goniometry. *Physical Therapy Review.* 1949;29(Pt 3):302.

Higbie EJ, Seidel-Cobb D, Taylor LF, Cummings GS. Effect of head position on vertical mandibular opening. *J Orthop Sports Phys Ther.* 1999;29(2): 127-130.

Hoppenfeld S. *Physical Examination of the Spine and Extremities.* New York, NY: Appleton-Century-Crofts; 1976.

Hopson MM, McPoil TG, Cornwall MW. Motion of the first metatarsophalangeal joint. Reliability and validity of four measurement techniques. *Journal of the American Podiatric Medical Association.* 1995;85(4):198-204.

Hollis M, Yung P. *Patient Examination and Assessment for Therapists.* Boston, MA: Blackwell Scientific Publications; 1985.

Kapandji IA. *The Physiology of the Joints.* 5th ed. Vol. 1. Upper Limb. New York, NY: Churchill Livingstone; 1982.

Kapandji IA. *The Physiology of the Joints.* 5th ed. Vol. 2. Lower Limb. New York, NY: Churchill Livingstone; 1987.

Kendall FP, Kendall HO, Wadsworth GE. *Muscle Testing and Function.* 2nd ed. Baltimore, MD: Williams and Wilkins; 1971.

Krusen FH, Kottke FJ, Ellwood PM. *Handbook of Physical Medicine and Rehabilitation.* 2nd ed. Philadelphia, PA: WB Saunders; 1971.

Levangie P, Norkin C. *Joint Structure and Function: A Comprehensive Analysis.* 3rd ed. Philadelphia, PA: FA Davis; 2001.

Magee DJ, Zachazewski JE, Quillen WS. *Scientific Principles of Practice in Musculoskeletal Rehabilitation.* St. Louis, MO: Saunders Elsevier; 2007.

Mallon WJ, Brown H, Nunley JA. Digital ranges of motion: normal values in young adults. *Journal of Hand Surgery.* 1991;16A (5): 882-887.

Moore ML. The measurement of joint motion: part II—the technic of goniometry. *Physical Therapy Review.* 1949;29(6):256-264.

Norkin CC, White DJ. *Measurement of Joint Motion.* 2nd ed. Philadelphia, PA: FA Davis; 1995.

O'Sullivan SB, Schmitz TJ. *Physical Rehabilitation.* 5th ed. Philadelphia, PA: FA Davis; 2007.

Palmer LM, Epler ME. *Clinical Assessment Procedures in Physical Therapy.* Philadelphia, PA: JB Lippincott; 1990.

Palmer LM, Epler ME. *Fundamentals of Musculoskeletal Techniques.* 2nd ed. Philadelphia, PA: Lippincott-Raven Publishers; 1998.

Piva SR, Fitzgerald K, Irrgang, JJ, Hando SJ, Browder DA, Childs JD. Reliability of measures of impairments associated with patellofemoral pain syndrome. *BMC Musculoskeletal Disorders.* 2006;7: 33.

Prentice WE, Voight ML. *Techniques in Musculoskeletal Rehabilitation.* New York, NY: McGraw-Hill; 2001.

Reynolds PMG. Measurement of spinal mobility: a comparison of three methods. *Rheumatology and Rehabilitation.* 1975;14:180-185.

Roaas A, Anderson GBJ. Normal range of motion of the hip, knee and ankle joints in male subjects, 30-40 years of age. *Acta Orthopaedica.* 1982;53(2): 205-208.

Roach KE, Miles TP. Normal hip and knee active range of motion: the relationship to age. *Phys Ther.* 1991;71(9):656-664.

Rothstein JM. *Measurement in Physical Therapy.* New York, NY: Churchill Livingstone; 1985.

Salter N. Methods of measurement of muscle and joint function. *J Bone Joint Surg Br.* 1955;34:474.

Schenker AW. Goniometry—an improved method of joint measurement. *New York State Journal of Medicine.* 1956;56(4): 539-545.

Smith LK, Weiss EL, Lehmkuhl DL. *Brunnstrom's Clinical Kinesiology.* 5th ed. Philadelphia, PA: FA Davis; 1996.

Van Ost L. *Goniometry.* Thorofare, NJ: SLACK Incorporated; 1999.

Walker N, Bohannon RW, Cameron D. Discriminant validity of temporomandibular joint range of motion measurements obtained with a ruler. *J Orthop Sports Phys Ther.* 2000;30(8):484-492.

Watkins MA, Riddle DL, Lamb RL, Personius WJ. Reliability of goniometric measurements and visual estimates of knee range of motion obtained in a clinical setting. *Phys Ther.* 1991;71(2):90-97.

West CC. Measurement of joint motion. *Arch Phys Med Rehabil.* 1945;26:414.

Youdas JW, Carey JR, Garrett TR. Reliability of measurements of cervical spine range of motion—comparison of three methods. *Phys Ther.* 1991;71(2):98-104.

Youdas JW, Garrett TR, Suman VJ, Bogard CL, Hallman HO, Carey JR. Normal range of motion of the cervical spine: an initial goniometric study. *Phys Ther.* 1992;72(11):770-780.

INDEX

anatomical zero, 168–169
ankle, 116–119
    dorsiflexion, 116–117
    normal range of motion, 166–167
    plantarflexion, 118–119

carpometacarpal joint, 68–77
    abduction, 72–73
    adduction, 74–75
    extension, 70–71
    flexion, 68–69
    opposition, 76–77
cervical spine, 1–9
    extension, 4–5
    flexion, 2–3
    hyperextension, 4–5
    lateral flexion, 6–7
    rotation, 8–9

digits, normal range of motion, 164–165
distal interphalangeal joint, 64–67, 146–149
    extension, 66–67, 148–149
    flexion, 64–65, 146–147

elbow, 36–39
    extension, 38–39
    flexion, 36–37
    normal range of motion, 164–165

fingers-digits II to V, 52–67
    abduction, 56–57
    adduction, 58–59
    extension, 54–55, 62–63, 66–67
    flexion, 52–53, 60–61, 64–65
    hyperextension, 54–55
first toe, 128–137
    abduction, 132–133
    extension, 130–131, 136–137
    flexion, 128–129, 134–135
    hyperextension, 130–131, 136–137
    normal range of motion, 166–167
forearm, 40–43
    pronation, 40–41
    supination, 42–43

glenohumeral joint, 20–35
    abduction, 24–25
    adduction, 26–27
    extension, 22–23
    external lateral rotation, 34–35
    flexion, 20–21
    horizontal abduction, 28–29
    horizontal adduction, 30–31
    hyperextension, 22–23
    internal medial rotation, 32–33
goniometric measurement, procedure for, 160

hindfoot, 120–123
    eversion, 122–123
    inversion, 120–121
hip, 98–109
    abduction, 102–103
    adduction, 104–105

extension, 100–101
    external (lateral) rotation, 108–109
    flexion, 98–99
    hyperextension, 100–101
    internal (medial) rotation, 106–107
    normal range of motion, 166–167
humeroradial joint, 36–39
    extension, 38–39
    flexion, 36–37
humeroulnar joint, 36–39
    extension, 38–39
    flexion, 36–37

intercarpal joint, 44–51
    extension, 46–47
    flexion, 44–45
    hyperextension, 46–47
    radial deviation abduction, 48–49
    ulnar deviation adduction, 50–51
interphalangeal joint, 82–85, 134–137
    distal, 64–67, 146–149
        extension, 66–67, 148–149
        flexion, 64–65, 146–147
    extension, 84–85, 136–137
    flexion, 82–83, 134–135
    hyperextension, 84–85, 136–137
    proximal, 142–145
        extension, 144–145
        flexion, 142–143

knee, 110–113
    extension, 112–113
    flexion, 110–111
    normal range of motion, 166–167

lateral toes, 138–149
    extension, 140–141, 144–145, 148–149
    flexion, 138–139, 142–143, 146–147
    hyperextension, 140–141
lower extremity, 97–149
    ankle, 116–119
        dorsiflexion, 116–117
        plantarflexion, 118–119
    distal interphalangeal joint, 146–149
        extension, 148–149
        flexion, 146–147
    first toe (interphalangeal joint), 134–137
        extension, 136–137
        flexion, 134–135
        hyperextension, 136–137
    first toe (metatarsophalangeal joint),
        128–133
        abduction, 132–133
        extension, 130–131
        flexion, 128–129
        hyperextension, 130–131
    hindfoot, 120–123
        eversion, 122–123
        inversion, 120–121
    hip, 98–109
        abduction, 102–103
        adduction, 104–105

extension, 100–101
external (lateral) rotation, 108–109
flexion, 98–99
hyperextension, 100–101
internal (medial) rotation, 106–107
interphalangeal joint, 134–137
extension, 136–137
flexion, 134–135
hyperextension, 136–137
knee (tibiofemoral joint), 110–113
extension, 112–113
flexion, 110–111
lateral toes (distal interphalangeal joints), 146–149
extension, 148–149
flexion, 146–147
lateral toes (metatarsophalangeal joints), 138–141
extension, 140–141
flexion, 138–139
hyperextension, 140–141
lateral toes (proximal interphalangeal joints), 142–145
extension, 144–145
flexion, 142–143
metatarsophalangeal joint, 128–133, 138–141
abduction, 132–133
extension, 130–131, 140–141
flexion, 128–129, 138–139
hyperextension, 130–131, 140–141
midtarsal joint, 124–127
eversion, 126–127
inversion, 124–125
proximal interphalangeal joint, 142–145
extension, 144–145
flexion, 142–143
subtalar joint (hindfoot), 120–123
eversion, 122–123
inversion, 120–121
tibial, torsion, 114–115
tibiofemoral joint, 110–113
extension, 112–113
flexion, 110–111
transverse tarsal (midtarsal) joint, 124–127
eversion, 126–127
inversion, 124–125
lumbar spine, 87–95
thoracolumbar extension, 90–91
thoracolumbar flexion, 88–89
thoracolumbar hyperextension, 90–91
thoracolumbar lateral flexion, 92–93
thoracolumbar rotation, 94–95
thoracolumbar spine, 88–95

mandible, 152–157
anterior protrusion of, 154–155
depression of (opening of mouth), 152–153
lateral protrusion of, 156–157
metacarpophalangeal joint, 52–59, 78–81
abduction, 56–57
adduction, 58–59
extension, 54–55, 80–81
flexion, 52–53, 78–79
hyperextension, 54–55, 80–81
metatarsophalangeal joint, 128–133, 138–141

abduction, 132–133
extension, 130–131, 140–141
flexion, 128–129, 138–139
hyperextension, 130–131, 140–141
midtarsal joint, 124–127
eversion, 126–127
inversion, 124–125
mouth, opening of, 152–153

normal range of motion values, adults, 164–167

opening of mouth, 152–153

procedure for goniometric measurement, 160
proximal interphalangeal joint, 60–63, 142–145
extension, 62–63, 144–145
flexion, 60–61, 142–143

radiocarpal joint, 44–51
extension, 46–47
flexion, 44–45
hyperextension, 46–47
radial deviation abduction, 48–49
ulnar deviation adduction, 50–51
radioulnar joint, 40–43
normal range of motion, 164–165
pronation, 40–41
supination, 42–43
range of motion values, adults, 164–167

scapulothoracic joint, 12–19
abduction, 16–17
adduction, 18–19
downward rotation, 14–15
upward rotation, 12–13
shoulder, 20–35
abduction, 24–25
adduction, 26–27
extension, 22–23
external (lateral) rotation, 34–35
flexion, 20–21
horizontal abduction, 28–29
horizontal adduction, 30–31
hyperextension, 22–23
internal (medial) rotation, 32–33
normal range of motion, 164–165
spine, cervical, 1–9
extension, 4–5
flexion, 2–3
hyperextension, 4–5
lateral flexion, 6–7
rotation, 8–9
subtalar joint, 120–123
eversion, 122–123
inversion, 120–121
normal range of motion, 166–167

temporomandibular joint, 151–157
anterior protrusion of mandible, 154–155
depression of mandible (opening of mouth), 152–153
lateral protrusion of mandible, 156–157
thoracic spine, 87–95
extension, 90–91
flexion, 88–89
hyperextension, 90–91

lateral flexion, 92–93
    rotation, 94–95
thoracolumbar extension, 90–91
thoracolumbar flexion, 88–89
thoracolumbar hyperextension, 90–91
thoracolumbar lateral flexion, 92–93
thoracolumbar rotation, 94–95
thoracolumbar spine, 88–95
thumb, 68–85
    abduction, 72–73
    adduction, 74–75
    extension, 70–71, 80–81, 84–85
    flexion, 68–69, 78–79, 82–83
    hyperextension, 80–81, 84–85
    normal range of motion, 164–165
    opposition, 76–77
tibial, torsion, 114–115
tibiofemoral joint, 110–113
    extension, 112–113
    flexion, 110–111
TMJ joint. See temporomandibular joint
toes, normal range of motion, 166–167
transverse tarsal joint, 124–127
    eversion, 126–127
    inversion, 124–125
    normal range of motion, 166–167

universal goniometer, 162
upper extremity, 11–85
    carpometacarpal joint, 68–77
        abduction, 72–73
        adduction, 74–75
        extension, 70–71
        flexion, 68–69
        opposition, 76–77
    distal interphalangeal joint, 64–67
        extension, 66–67
        flexion, 64–65
    elbow, 36–39
        extension, 38–39
        flexion, 36–37
    fingers-digits II to V, 52–67
        abduction, 56–57
        adduction, 58–59
        extension, 54–55, 62–63, 66–67
        flexion, 52–53, 60–61, 64–65
        hyperextension, 54–55
    forearm, 40–43
        pronation, 40–41
        supination, 42–43
    glenohumeral joint, 20–35
        abduction, 24–25
        adduction, 26–27
        extension, 22–23
        external lateral rotation, 34–35
        flexion, 20–21
        horizontal abduction, 28–29
        horizontal adduction, 30–31
        hyperextension, 22–23
        internal medial rotation, 32–33
    humeroradial joint, 36–39
        extension, 38–39
        flexion, 36–37
    humeroulnar joint, 36–39
        extension, 38–39
        flexion, 36–37

intercarpal joint, 44–51
    extension, 46–47
    flexion, 44–45
    hyperextension, 46–47
    radial deviation abduction, 48–49
    ulnar deviation adduction, 50–51
interphalangeal joint, 82–85
    extension, 84–85
    flexion, 82–83
    hyperextension, 84–85
metacarpophalangeal joint, 52–59, 78–81
    abduction, 56–57
    adduction, 58–59
    extension, 54–55, 80–81
    flexion, 52–53, 78–79
    hyperextension, 54–55, 80–81
proximal interphalangeal joint, 60–63
    extension, 62–63
    flexion, 60–61
radiocarpal joint, 44–51
    extension, 46–47
    flexion, 44–45
    hyperextension, 46–47
    radial deviation abduction, 48–49
    ulnar deviation adduction, 50–51
radioulnar joint, 40–43
    pronation, 40–41
    supination, 42–43
scapulothoracic joint, 12–19
    abduction, 16–17
    adduction, 18–19
    downward rotation, 14–15
    upward rotation, 12–13
shoulder, 20–35
    abduction, 24–25
    adduction, 26–27
    extension, 22–23
    external (lateral) rotation, 34–35
    flexion, 20–21
    horizontal abduction, 28–29
    horizontal adduction, 30–31
    hyperextension, 22–23
    internal (medial) rotation, 32–33
thumb, 68–85
    abduction, 72–73
    adduction, 74–75
    extension, 70–71, 80–81, 84–85
    flexion, 68–69, 78–79, 82–83
    hyperextension, 80–81, 84–85
    opposition, 76–77
wrist, 44–51
    extension, 46–47
    flexion, 44–45
    hyperextension, 46–47
    radial deviation (abduction), 48–49
    ulnar deviation (adduction), 50–51

wrist, 44–51
    extension, 46–47
    flexion, 44–45
    hyperextension, 46–47
    normal range of motion, 164–165
    radial deviation (abduction), 48–49
    ulnar deviation (adduction), 50–51

zero, anatomical, 168–169

Wait...There's More!

SLACK Incorporated's Health Care Books and Journals offers a wide selection of books in the field of Athletic Training. We are dedicated to providing important works that educate, inform, and improve the knowledge of our customers. Don't miss out on our other informative titles that will enhance your collection.

Special Tests for Orthopedic Examination, Third Edition

Jeff G. Konin PhD, ATC, PT; Denise L. Wiksten PhD, ATC; Jerome A. Isear, Jr. MS, PT, ATC-L; Holly Brader MPH, RN, BSN, ATC

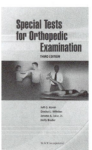

400 pp, Soft Cover, 2006, ISBN 13 978-1-55642-741-1, Order# 47417, $43.95

Special Tests for Orthopedic Examination has been used for over 10 years by thousands of students, clinicians, and rehab professionals and is now available in a revised and updated *Third Edition*. Concise and pocket-sized, this handbook is an invaluable guide filled with the most current and practical clinical exam techniques used during an orthopedic examination. Students, clinicians, and rehabilitation professionals alike will benefit from adding this classic text to their reference library today.

Special Tests for Neurologic Examination

James R. Scifers DScPT, PT, SCS, LAT, ATC

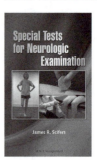

432 pp, Soft Cover, 2008, ISBN 13 978-155642-797-8, Order# 47972, $43.95

Ideal for students and clinicians to access quick clinical information, *Special Tests for Neurologic Examination* offers invaluable evaluation and assessment tips and techniques for neurologic conditions commonly found in patients. Organized in an easy-to-use format, this book is the perfect guide for practicing clinical skills and reviewing for licensure and certification examinations.

Please visit **www.slackbooks.com** to order any of the above titles!
24 Hours a Day...7 Days a Week!

Attention Industry Partners!

Whether you are interested in buying multiple copies of a book, chapter reprints, or looking for something new and different — we are able to accommodate your needs.

MULTIPLE COPIES

At attractive discounts starting for purchases as low as 25 copies for a single title, SLACK Incorporated will be able to meet all your of your needs.

CHAPTER REPRINTS

SLACK Incorporated is able to offer the chapters you want in a format that will lead to success. Bound with an attractive cover, use the chapters that are a fit specifically for your company Available for quantities of 100 or more.

CUSTOMIZE

SLACK Incorporated is able to create a specialized custom version of any of our products specifically for your company.

Please contact the Marketing Communications Director for further details on multiple copy purchases, chapter reprints or custom printing at 1-800-257-8290 or 1-856-848-1000.

*Please note all conditions are subject to change.

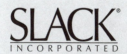